A beginner's

the rc ... ts
of yoga

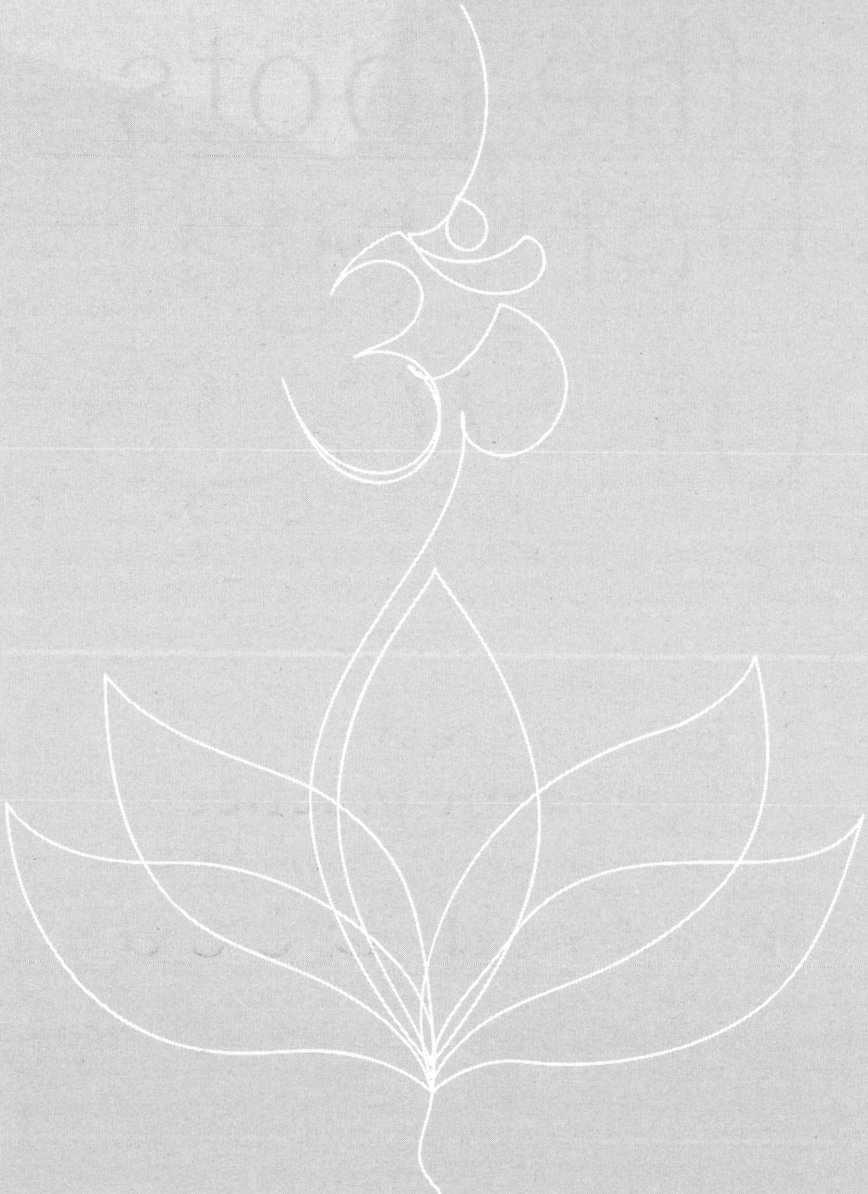

A beginner's guide to the roots of yoga

How to create a more authentic practice

Nikita Desai

GREEN TREE
LONDON • OXFORD • NEW YORK • NEW DELHI • SYDNEY

GREEN TREE
Bloomsbury Publishing Plc
50 Bedford Square, London, WC1B 3DP, UK
29 Earlsfort Terrace, Dublin 2, Ireland

BLOOMSBURY, GREEN TREE and the Green Tree logo are trademarks of Bloomsbury Publishing Plc

First published in Great Britain 2025

A catalogue record for this book is available from the British Library.

Library of Congress Cataloguing-in-Publication data has been applied for.

ISBN: TPB: 978-1-3994-1110-3; eBook: 978-1-3994-1109-7; ePdf: 978-1-3994-1111-0

2 4 6 8 10 9 7 5 3 1

Text design by Austin Taylor
Illustrations on pp. 144, 148, 197, 198, 202, 205, 209 by Barking Dog Art

Plate section images are author's own with the exception of: Page 1, bottom: @yogandphoto; Page 2, bottom left: Getty Images; Page 4, Getty Images; Page 5, Shutterstock; Page 6, Top left: ©R.H. Meadow/Harappa.com, Courtesy Dept. of Archaeology and Museums, Govt. of Pakistan, bottom: Getty Images; Page 7, top and bottom left: Getty Images, bottom right: Shutterstock; Page 8: @yogandphoto

Typeset in Avenir Next and Kohinoor by Deanta Global Publishing Services, Chennai, India
Printed and bound in Great Britain by CPI Group (UK) Ltd., Croydon, CR0 4YY

FSC www.fsc.org MIX Paper | Supporting responsible forestry FSC® C171272

For my parents, whose love, support, and encouragement will always be carried in my heart. A special mention to my sister, who has not just been a sibling but also one of my greatest mentors and protectors, embodying a nurturing presence in my life.

And for my little fur girl, Kali, whose presence has been a constant source of comfort with every word penned (or typed!). Those solitary writing moments will always be cherished because of you.

A note on the text

Please note that *A Beginner's Guide to the Roots of Yoga* reflects my own understanding and interpretation of yoga, but do bear in mind that there are many interpretations out there. Also, I've used suitable language for the time of writing, but it's important to recognise that language evolves over time. Finally, this book may spark as many questions for you as it provides answers, and that's OK. Feel free to jot down any questions that arise as you go so you can explore these further in your own time. I am a forever pupil of yoga and I invite you to be so, too.

Contents

Foreword

Vex King

It seems that nowadays, you can't scroll through social media without encountering a reference to yoga. More often than not, these posts showcase individuals in impossibly flexible poses set against stunning backdrops. While visually captivating, this portrayal barely scratches the surface of yoga's profound depth and rich heritage.

In this landscape of filtered yoga reality, Nikita Desai's *A Beginner's Guide to the Roots of Yoga* emerges as a refreshing oasis of authenticity and wisdom. Having observed and experienced the transformation of yoga in the West over recent years, I can't emphasise enough how crucial and timely this work is.

My own journey with yoga has been metamorphic, evolving from a mere physical practice to a profound philosophical guide for life. Over the years, I've come to understand that yoga, in its truest sense, means 'union' – a harmonious integration of mind, body, and spirit. It's not just about mastering poses but about mastering oneself.

The ancient wisdom of yoga has been my compass through both calm and stormy seas. It has taught me to find balance amidst the chaos, to breathe through challenges, and to cultivate a sense of inner peace even when the world around me is in turmoil.

Furthermore, yoga's teachings on mindfulness have sharpened my awareness, allowing me to live more fully in the present moment.

Its emphasis on self-study (**svādhyāya**) has led me to profound self-discovery, helping me understand my conditioned patterns, overcome limitations, and tap into my innate potential. The principle of non-attachment (**vairāgya**) has been particularly powerful, inspiring me to let go of what no longer serves me and to find contentment in the present.

With clarity and reverence, Desai takes us on a journey back to the true essence of yoga. She skilfully unveils the layers of this ancient practice, from its historical origins to its spiritual significance, in a way that is both accessible to beginners and enlightening for seasoned practitioners. Her exploration of the four key **mārgas** of yoga – **Karma**, **Bhakti**, **Rāja** and **Jñāna** – provides a comprehensive framework for understanding yoga as a holistic path to self-realisation.

What sets this book apart is Desai's relentless commitment to presenting yoga in its most authentic form. She doesn't shy away from addressing the issues of cultural appropriation and commercialisation that have become prevalent in modern yoga. Instead, she offers a thoughtful critique and a pathway back to respectful, mindful practice.

I found myself particularly moved by Desai's discussion of yoga's potential for personal growth. Her insights into how traditional yoga practices can be applied to navigate the challenges of modern life are both practical and profound. As I read, I was reminded of my own moments of revelation beyond the mat – times when a simple breath opened up new realms of self-understanding.

Desai's writing style is a testament to her deep knowledge and passion for the subject. She manages to convey complex concepts with remarkable clarity, making the esoteric accessible without oversimplification. Her voice is that of a knowledgeable friend, guiding the reader with patience and enthusiasm.

This body of text is more than just a book; it's an invitation to embark on an evolutionary journey. Whether you're new to yoga or have been practising for years, Desai's work will deepen your understanding and enrich your practice. It serves as a much-needed bridge between the ancient wisdom of yoga and our modern lives, reminding us that the true power of yoga lies not in perfecting poses, but in cultivating inner peace and self-awareness.

As you turn these pages, I encourage you to approach them with an open heart and mind. Allow Desai's words to challenge your preconceptions and inspire you to explore the depths of this timeless practice. In doing so, you'll not only gain a richer understanding of yoga but also of yourself.

In a world that often feels disconnected and chaotic, Nikita Desai's book is a gentle reminder of the transformative power of authentic yoga. I sincerely believe this work will educate, inspire, and play a crucial role in preserving and promoting the true spirit of yoga for future generations.

Vex King, July 2024

Introduction

Would you like to know more about yoga, but don't know where to start? Well, you're in the right place. Whether you're a complete beginner to yoga or a seasoned practitioner looking to learn more, this is the book for you. My goal is to give you the essential toolkit to help you establish a respectful and authentic yoga practice, so you can enjoy the benefits that come from embracing this ancient practice in its full and true form while also ensuring you are a responsible practitioner along the way.

Why is this book needed?

Before we get started, I think it's important to consider why a beginner's guide to traditional yoga is still needed, despite yoga having been popular for so long. As I see it, there are three key reasons why this outline of yoga is required. Let's discuss them.

First, although yoga has become popular in the Western world, this mainstream form of 'yoga' that we've become accustomed to actually looks very different from yoga in its authentic form. If you think of yoga like a pie (bear with me on this...), then the West has largely fixated on one tiny slice of the whole 'yoga pie': the physical yoga poses. This unbalanced focus gives unnecessary prominence to these, and unfortunately means that the majority of yoga's other traditional teachings and benefits (i.e. the rest of the 'pie') have largely become lost along the way. Yoga in its 'full' or traditional form goes beyond the mat and involves deep self-reflection and a lifestyle that, if done correctly, can benefit us not only as individuals but as a collective, too.

Second, with an undue focus on physical poses in Western yoga comes a needless fixation on a practitioner's flexibility, fitness level and physical appearance, which can impact their ability to access yoga spaces comfortably. Modern yoga spaces are typically dominated by women who are white, slim, able-bodied and wearing certain clothing, which can make many of us who do not fit within this particular mould feel excluded. This outcome is completely at odds with the traditional inclusive teachings of authentic yoga. I know of ways that every single person can practise yoga, regardless of shape, size, flexibility, race, gender or social class, and I see the demand for accessible and inclusive practices becoming more and more apparent. Learning about yoga in its authentic form is therefore important because it helps us uphold the element of inclusivity that is at yoga's core and allows more people to access the practice.

Finally, for those of us who wish to learn more about traditional yoga (and I know there are many!), the resources currently available to support this learning are limited. The teachings of yoga are written in classical languages, such as Sanskrit (see p. 26), meaning there is very little information readily available in English. Many of the English resources that are available can be dense and inaccessible or are poor translations of the original teachings. This can leave the most well-meaning practitioner feeling overwhelmed when attempting to research yoga on their own, or vulnerable to unknowingly digesting and passing on misinformation.

The good news, though, is that while I've been on my own personal yoga journey (more on this next), I've seen the amazing appetite that there is in the Western world for more information about authentic yoga. The even better news is that I've done the hard work for you of going through the key parts of ancient texts myself, so I am now able to guide you through the basics of what I have learned (and – as an aside – of what I am continuing to learn, because, as you'll soon discover, the path to learning is never-ending when it comes to yoga!). I have found ways to make the ancient teachings accessible and digestible so that practitioners, just like you, can truly benefit from what authentic yoga has to offer.

So, whatever your reason for being here, I'm glad that you are. It's great that you're open to learning more about yoga in its traditional form, whatever stage you're currently at in your own practice. Whether you're a complete beginner or a practising teacher, I promise you that the knowledge in this book will only help deepen your practice. Yes, yoga in its Western form can be an entry point and have benefits, but I can assure you that the more you align your practice with the authentic teachings of traditional yoga, the more you will benefit from it.

I'd like to make it clear from the start that if you already have an established yoga practice then I am not suggesting you forget this: after all, it has most likely benefitted you in many ways. But the teachings we'll discuss here will certainly help to enhance your current practice. Or, if you're completely new to yoga, then the information that we'll explore together in this book will help you set up foundations steeped in authentic teachings right from the off. Starting out with yoga should never feel intimidating and it's a journey that can begin with a few simple steps, so whether you are sitting in a chair or lying on a bed, I'm excited to explore this together.

My journey with yoga

You may be wondering who I am and how I got to the point of writing this book, so let me introduce myself and explain my own journey with yoga before we go any further.

Yoga as a child

I am of Hindu heritage and my family are from Gujarat on the western coast of India. Despite being born and raised in the UK, my family life is rooted in my Hindu heritage and my connection to India has always remained strong. This is thanks to the cherished traditions that were passed down by my parents and grandparents. Visits to India, beginning when I was very young, helped to deepen my understanding of my roots, and spending time with family in Gujarat created memories that form an important part of my cultural narrative.

From a very young age I was introduced to yoga in the form of meditative practices focused on the mind and through **mantras** (sacred chants performed in Sanskrit). The practice never involved fancy clothing or equipment (and certainly didn't require breaking a sweat!). Instead, the lighting of **diyas** (oil lamps) and chanting of **mantras** in the morning and evening symbolised a connection to a higher power and a way of cultivating stillness. Visits to my grandparents during the weekends or holidays meant following their routine, which involved writing down these sacred **mantras** multiple times as a form of meditation. These practices encouraged us to turn inwards and were centred on our devotion to Hindu deities.

This practice of yoga that I have just described was deeply embedded in me but, as with most Hindus, I had very little awareness that it was a form of yoga. These rituals, traditions and practices that are carried out in our culture are so ingrained in our upbringing that we live yoga through our daily actions without questioning them. It was only much later on that I learned that these rituals – practised by almost all my family members – were linked to the meanings of yoga (as we'll be exploring in **Part 3**).

Yoga in the Western world

My personal pursuit of yoga in the Western world began much later, when I was in my early twenties. I say 'yoga in the Western world' because the yoga practised in the Western world felt quite different to my experience of yoga in my family home. So different, in fact, that when I was initially reintroduced to yoga from a Western perspective, I did not immediately recognise its connection to the rituals of my childhood. I understood that 'yoga' in the West had an Indian background, but I saw Western yoga and my childhood practices as two entirely different things. Let me explain.

In 2014, a significant event occurred in my life: I sustained an unfortunate lumbar spine fracture during a skydiving experience. This injury in my lower back caused me agony and distress and, after numerous medical appointments, pain management and advice from different specialists and doctors, I received the news that the only way to heal was by having major surgery. Following advice from my doctor, I opted to explore holistic healing methods alongside conventional medical treatments for my condition (known as spondylolytic spondylolisthesis).

A few friends recommended yoga to me and, from a physical standpoint, it was not something that I had ever participated in. So, at the age of 26, I had my first encounter with **āsana** (Sanskrit for 'physical poses'). Stepping into what I thought of as completely unknown territory, I began practising **āsana** with the help of YouTube videos. It wasn't long before I felt the benefits, not just physically but mentally, too.

Mental health is something I have struggled with throughout my life. At the age of eight I was diagnosed with anxiety and severe depression and my symptoms remained severe until around the age of 10. Those symptoms then fluctuated throughout my teens and became worse as I got older. Throughout the years, I found it difficult to cope with intense periods of clinical depression, which the people closest to me never fully understood (as with so many others at the time, they simply weren't aware of mental health issues and their impacts). I saw therapists and doctors but my mental health was a constant challenge, and I was always trying to find a way to reduce the symptoms that it caused. Then, finally, beginning to practise Western-style yoga at the time of my back injury seemed to do exactly that. I started dedicating time to my practice twice a week and I even created a class schedule for myself that included more challenging postures like backbends, splits and inversions. These were the postures that I felt would be considered huge achievements if I could eventually master them.

At first, I didn't understand how these YouTube videos on physical exercises were helping my mind. However, as I dedicated myself to regular practice, my interest in learning more about the ways that I could heal myself using yoga grew. I found that through practising Western yoga, even over just a short period of time, I was able to adopt a much calmer state in stressful situations and to manage the pain that my back injury caused me. I quickly became curious about how such enormous effects could be experienced from a practice that required nothing but myself (i.e. my mind and my body). But I found that none of this was explained to me by my yoga teachers, either those that I learned from online or even in studio environments. The spiritual and philosophical aspects of yoga were seldom spoken about.

Keen for answers, I made it my aim to dig deeper into yoga – going beyond my focus on it as a physical practice – so that I could try to understand its healing aspects and share this information with others. Around this time, I was made redundant from my corporate job, and the opportunity to partake in a yoga teacher training course seemed to land at the right moment. My excitement took over while looking for a location in which to train. However, I was unable to find a course in my location of preference – India, the birthplace of yoga – so I chose to book myself on to a four-week, 200-hour training course in Thailand instead.*

As my training commenced, I started to notice a few aspects that didn't align with my expectations. One instance was the way **mantras** were being taught. It was at this point – through the teaching of **mantras** – that I finally understood that the yoga being taught in the Western world mirrored the yoga I had grown up with in my childhood. Through the course, these **mantras** were being passed on to large groups of practitioners by yoga teachers who weren't deeply rooted in the practice, by which I mean that the teachers were making mistakes. This was evident as the teachers' pronunciation wasn't always accurate, which likely arose from their lack of exposure to authentic sources and/or not having received accurate training themselves.

Mistakes stood out for me in one **mantra** in particular, the *Gāyatrī Mantra* (one of the most significant mantras in the **Vedas**†), because it is a **mantra** that still echoes in my mother's voice in my head. My mother would repeatedly sing this **mantra** to me as a lullaby when I was a child. It is also a **mantra** that I still use to soothe myself to sleep, and is very powerful if practised correctly. In Sanskrit, it's important that the words

* Two hundred hours is the standard qualification for yoga teachers. Some students, like me, choose to go on an intensive four-week course (often abroad) whereas some might complete their quota of hours over a longer course. It is relatively straightforward to become qualified; you can't really fail – a fact that can contribute to teachers with limited understanding of yogic philosophy, anatomy and other important aspects being allowed to teach classes.

† The term **Veda** means 'knowledge'. The **Vedas** are the oldest and most sacred body of texts that form the foundation of Hinduism and are considered the ultimate source of knowledge and wisdom. They are a collection of scriptures that were composed in India thousands of years ago. But the **Vedas** aren't made up of human knowledge; the knowledge in the **Vedas** comes from the spiritual world. The foundations of yoga as a path to self-discovery and self-realisation are interwoven through the teachings of the **Vedas**.

are pronounced correctly because the language is designed so that the sounds of the words carry the words' meaning (more on this on p. 27). Upon raising my concerns about the mispronounced Sanskrit terms with one of the lead teachers I was met with an apology. However, the next morning, the incorrect chanting continued, completely dismissing the fact that the teaching was incorrect.

Another observation that I made was that the only Indian teacher was a philosophy lecturer, and it was he alone who delivered all the training on the most important part of yoga (by which I mean yogic philosophy, which we'll discuss in **Part 3**). I found this hard to sit with. It was clear that the other teachers didn't want to, or were unable to, teach these elements of yoga in depth. Therefore, a teacher from India was employed but only given space to speak on the more difficult subjects, which really should be embedded in every teacher. I carried out the remainder of my training without speaking up again. I was confused and unsettled by my experience although I remained committed to my Western yoga journey, nonetheless. Therefore, once I returned home, my goal was to bag a regular gig at a studio in London and begin teaching.

Back in London, I soon became disheartened. I was struggling to find regular teaching jobs to enable me to make a living from yoga, but at the same time I saw so many yoga teachers (who I followed through my social media accounts) achieving this same goal. I soon recognised a pattern in the studios and brands that I contacted and came to the realisation that I didn't fit their preferred aesthetic. To be able to teach at a top studio or work with a well-known yoga brand, I would have to adopt the mould of being white, slender, established and super able-bodied (which I wasn't due to my back injury). This made me feel like I needed to work harder at becoming more flexible to fit this narrative as best as I could, and I soon began pushing my body past its limits, which resulted in a decline in my mental and physical health. I made achieving advanced postures the pinnacle of my learning since I thought that if I couldn't teach these then my place as a teacher was invalid.

Let's take stock for a moment here. At this time in my life, my understanding of Western yoga was as follows:

- Yoga is a physical practice.
- Flexibility is a must.

- The goal is to be able to perform the splits or an inversion.
- Every great yoga teacher/practitioner needs to be extremely toned, strong and fit.
- Yoga poses are separate from other elements, such as yoga philosophy.

Now, I'm sure we can all agree that this list of requirements would be daunting for most of us, even for individuals who are physically fit and healthy. Imagine the added challenges faced by those of us with physical limitations, larger body sizes or those – like myself – who struggle with low self-esteem, anxiety or depression. The pressure to meet the expectations of this list can feel immense, and it was this that led me to set yoga goals for myself centred around advanced physical postures that weren't healthy for me. This was when the Western culture of 'yoga' began feeling too exclusionary for me. I recognised that I wasn't fitting the desired mould at the same time that I realised more firmly that I was looking for something beyond the surface-level physical poses I was currently practising.

A moment of introspection

As I tell you my story with yoga, I invite you to reflect on your own experiences by considering the questions below:

- Have you ever felt pressure to conform to certain standards in your yoga practice?
- Were there worries that almost held you back (or have held you back) from starting yoga? Do they still play a role today?
- Have you ever taken a moment to rethink how you approach yoga?
- Are there any aspects of yoga that have become more significant to you beyond the physical poses?

There is no right or wrong way of answering these. Or you might not have answers yet and that's absolutely OK. These questions are simply gentle prompts to spark reflection, helping you to begin to discover what you truly need or desire from your yoga practice.

Yoga and teaching on social media

On realising what was important to me (i.e. a practice beyond the physical poses), two things changed. First, I found myself diving deeper into the ancient texts and teachings of yoga. I felt a strong desire to learn directly from teachers who were deeply rooted in the source culture. This led me to actively seek out opportunities to engage with them, both through the books I was reading and in person. This exploration became a crucial part of my journey as both a yoga teacher and a dedicated student.

Second, at the same time, I began searching for a yoga space that focused on authenticity and had a connection to yoga's roots, but it seemed almost impossible to find. Unable to secure enough regular work as a yoga teacher, I had returned to my corporate job, but the pandemic brought about another redundancy for me in 2020. This became another turning point as I decided to take a leap and create a yoga studio to bring my vision to life. I wanted to create a yoga space that was truly inclusive for people of all backgrounds and abilities. My goal was to form a place where yoga could be learned without the weight of expectations or limitations.

Alongside running the studio, I soon began creating educational online content to bring authenticity to yoga through social media platforms. By this point I had been teaching yoga for a few years, but I had found very little online depicting what yoga is at its core. Practising yoga in the West, as we've discussed, has become common and the perception of yoga is often that it's an exercise used to increase flexibility. Online creators and teachers on social platforms often further distort our view of yoga by spotlighting advanced postures and expensive outfits, thereby showcasing a practice that many of us, as beginners, turn away from for fear of not fitting in. Yet yoga should never feel intimidating.

During all the lockdowns, at a time when keeping mentally healthy was essential, I saw just how much people would benefit from fundamental yogic practices. But it was advanced posture-based yogic practices (often for the purpose of aesthetics) that I found to be most prevalent online. I had a strong urge to make a change in the industry. I wanted to help bring to light the traditional pillars of yoga that aim to heal us mentally, emotionally and energetically through the physical and spiritual ancient teachings. I wanted to show people how to regulate their nervous system using yogic methods in order to improve mental health. I wanted to show how yoga can be used not only to gain physical strength but also to improve emotional and mental strength.

I therefore began posting online. I started with content about the origins of yoga, which I had learned about through my own research. I rarely saw this type of content online, but it's essential for practitioners to have this context for the practice to remain authentic. My first few pieces of content about the origins of yoga went viral and brought to light a vast number of people globally who expressed how they thought yoga was a practice made in the Western world by white women. I found this completely bewildering, but it also motivated me more than ever to keep teaching the truths of the practice. I was coming across people who were only aware of **āsana** (yoga's physical poses) and who believed that yoga was a practice used solely for the purpose of stretching or exercise. I also heard from people who were keen to learn more but had never known where to look for this information before. I spent the following months creating short videos explaining different yogic practices and their benefits for several mental health conditions. People found these effective in their personal practices, so I continued sharing them.

Running alongside these pieces of content were videos that challenged the status quo of Western yoga more generally, which some found unnerving. Mostly, however, people found that my content resonated with their own experiences with yoga in the Western world, and how excluded they had been made to feel due to the one-size-fits-all narrative that was being displayed in studios in real life and online. My social media accounts started growing as more and more people felt like my page was a comfortable and safe space on which to express their feelings of discomfort around the yoga and wellness industry. They had found a space to be curious and explore the deeper aspects of yoga, and where there is no such thing as asking a silly question.

I was being applauded for teaching authentically and making the practice of yoga inclusive. I received hundreds of comments from people who said they admired my strength in expressing my views on difficult topics, such as the systemic oppression that the BIPOC community face in today's wellness industry (more on this in **Part 1**). My social media accounts were inundated with messages from the public thanking me for my work and urging me to continue speaking and teaching, but at times this was really draining. I was at the front of the firing line for online 'trolls', which has and still does impact my mental health.

Seeing how much people appreciated the educational content that I provided gave me the strength to conduct workshops on the roots of yoga, which I also began presenting publicly at wellness festivals and online summits. Again, this touched people in ways that I never could have imagined. I was being told that my work was encouraging others to facilitate open conversations with colleagues; others were prompted to write their dissertations on topics that I teach; and others told me they started teaching their children yoga after hearing me speak on how inclusive the practice is! I am so grateful to every single person who has ever contacted me about my work. Your support has kept me going.

I am asked on a daily (and sometimes even hourly!) basis for more education on how to practise yoga authentically. Many individuals are eager to find a genuine starting point for their yoga journey, and people are seeking information that is preferably provided by someone from the source culture. This guide is an answer to all those questions and it's the book that I wish I had had when I began exploring yoga. It's designed to hold you through your yoga journey while encouraging you to practise respectfully, too. I do hope you enjoy it.

How to use this book

'Books are infinite in number, and time is short; therefore, this is the secret of knowledge, to take that which is essential.'

– *The Yoga Sūtras of Patañjali* by Swami Vivekananda

Since I've written this guide to be beginner-friendly, I have tried to keep a balance between being informative while not overwhelming you with too much detail. I also want to confess that it took me several attempts to work out where to start. I think this is important to mention for two main reasons.

First, my uncertainty over where to begin – and my hesitation over what to include – speaks to the sheer scale of the learnings available to us through yoga. It would be impossible for me (or anyone else) to cover *everything* in one book but, from my research, I have worked hard to design a roadmap of the absolute yoga essentials that I think you need to know when getting started. Therefore, please see this book as a jumping-off point from which you can continue your own research as/when needed. (I've included some ideas on how to continue your learning in **Part 4**, on p. 219.)

Second, my hesitation over where to begin demonstrates that if you ever feel stuck on your own yoga journey, or if you've ever felt stuck before, then know that you're not alone. With yoga it can often feel like the more you learn, the more you realise there is to learn. When I first began researching traditional yoga, I experienced much overwhelm and confusion … but don't let this put you off. As we'll discover, yoga is a life-long practice of self-discovery and the more you embrace the depth of the journey then the richer your journey will become. I see myself as a forever student in this practice and keeping this humility in mind helps me to embody traditional yoga in its full form (as we'll explore in **Part 3**). I invite you to adopt this same approach.

I also want to give a word of warning here. If you're only familiar with Western yoga, then there's a chance that learning about authentic yoga for the first time might feel quite uncomfortable at times. My advice to you is to go at the pace you need and to take comfort from the fact that by acknowledging uncomfortable discussions around yoga today, which are usually glossed over or omitted, you are putting yourself in the best possible position to honour and benefit from yoga as much as possible.

Also, if you're attached to your current Western yoga practice, then it might feel challenging to be asked to consider a new (to you!) traditional approach. I simply ask you to approach this book with the same open-mindedness that we aim for in our complete yoga practice. Even taking one or two steps towards making your current Western practice more inclusive and authentic is moving in the right direction, and that's a great start.

Likewise, any time you come across the terms 'God', 'universe' or 'the divine' in my writing, feel free to substitute them with whichever higher power resonates with your beliefs. Your personal connection to yoga matters.

For this same reason, keep an eye out for the 'Moments of introspection' sprinkled throughout. These moments hold a special place in our exploration as they will help you reflect on how our discussions relate to you personally. If jotting down your thoughts and feelings is challenging, simply take a few minutes to contemplate these questions for yourself or feel free to engage in a conversation with someone as they arise. Your insights are valuable, however you choose to express them.

From **Part 3** onwards, I introduce ways for you to start to practise authentic yoga. Look out for this symbol: . Practices with a sound symbol have an audio component; you can listen to me guiding these practices by going to bloomsbury.com/yogaaudio.

For many people, reading an entire book from start to finish can be a bit overwhelming, too. If that's you, then there's absolutely no pressure to read this all at once. If you prefer to pick it up, take what you need and return to it later, that's perfectly OK. If you're dipping in and out and encounter something that doesn't quite make sense though, then it's worth exploring the other sections of the book to find the answers and the context you need. But feel free to take from this book what you need and drop in and out as suits you.

Here's an outline of everything that we'll be covering:

Part 1: Why we should aim for an authentic yoga practice

We'll begin by contextualising the Western form of yoga as we know it today and discussing some of the issues that can arise with yoga in this current form. This will help us understand the benefits of adopting a more authentic yoga practice and why this work is so important.

Part 2: The foundations of yoga and a very brief history

We'll then move on to explore the roots, history and origins of yoga. Here we'll discuss the most pivotal moments in history and the key gurus and scriptures that laid the foundations for our practice today. Having this context will help shape your own practice and make it a more authentic one.

Part 3: Integrating authenticity into your practice

This is the practical section of the book as we'll look at how to begin to apply traditional teachings of yoga to your current practice (or show you how to begin your practice if you don't currently have one). In other words, we'll begin to study ourselves through yoga and learn how to centre key yogic principles and philosophy into our practice.

Part 4: Continuing your journey

Here we'll look at some of the ways you can continue your practice and learning if you'd like to explore further beyond this book.

Ready? Let's begin.

A note on Sanskrit

What is Sanskrit and why does using Sanskrit matter?

The principles and philosophy of yoga are written down in ancient Indian sacred texts, such as the **Vedas**, *The Yoga Sūtras of Patañjali* and the *Bhagavad Gita* (see **Part 2** for more), and the majority of these texts are written in the Sanskrit language. The word 'Sanskrit' is the English translation for the term **saṃskṛta**, which means 'refined' or 'perfected'. Sanskrit is known as **dēvavāṇī**, meaning the 'language of the Gods', and it is one of the main languages through which the wisdom of yoga has been passed down for thousands of years.*

Therefore, throughout this book, I will be using Sanskrit terms when I refer to yogic concepts, ideas or poses. These will be highlighted in bold text. You may be familiar with some Sanskrit terms already – such

* Sanskrit is *one* of the languages of yoga, but it's not the only language of yoga. Sanskrit is the one that has been used most widely though, so a lot of the yogic terms you will come across (if not all) will be written in the Sanskrit language, and that's what we'll focus on in this book.

as **āsana** meaning 'physical poses' – but others may be completely new to you. (There may even be some terms that you thought you knew the meaning of but which, in fact, have completely different connotations ... so watch out for those!)

Let me acknowledge now that Sanskrit, and yoga terminology in general, is not always easy to learn. But there are important reasons for making every effort to use the Sanskrit language in yoga spaces. I'll touch on two of the key reasons for you now:

1. **Preserving tradition** – Using Sanskrit in yoga helps to preserve the roots and cultural integrity of the ancient practice. You wouldn't pronounce ballet terms in any other language but French, right? So, in the same way, yoga without the use of Sanskrit (or the other languages that are associated with yoga) doesn't make much sense either! Using the correct Sanskrit language helps us stay connected to the deep history of yoga and keeps our practice authentic.
2. **Sounds and vibrations** – The Sanskrit terms that we use in yoga aren't just words; they're more than that. This is because the Sanskrit language is designed for the words, when pronounced correctly, to carry unique sounds and vibrations that hold extra meaning. Therefore, in Indian culture, it is believed that incorporating Sanskrit terms into our practice adds a further layer of depth to our yoga, as each Sanskrit term can influence the energetic aspects of our practice.

Pronunciation and common Sanskrit terms

My teacher Prasad Rangnekar has summarised some of the key components of the Sanskrit language:

> 'Sanskrit is a phonetic language and gives much importance to accents, pitch and pronunciation. It consists of 14 vowels and 33 consonants, and therefore the phonetics in Sanskrit are much broader than those of the English language. There are no silent letters. In Sanskrit, there is a one-to-one correspondence between words and pronunciation, unlike French or English. This is why precision in Sanskrit pronunciation is desirable as

it makes for clear communication and reduces the chances of being misunderstood.'

When reading Sanskrit words in books, you'll often notice diacritics, which are marks above or below letters. These diacritics help to distinguish meanings between words that might otherwise appear the same. For example, **nava** means 'nine', while **nāva** means 'boat or ship'. In this instance, **nava** would have a non-extended vowel while **nāva** would be pronounced 'naava', with the 'ā' as a long vowel, which completely changes the meaning.

In the Sanskrit language each term has equal stress, so stress emphasis does not feature in the same way as in English. The diacritics on vowels, though, which indicate longer sounds, are a helpful guide for English speakers to approach pronunciation e.g. **Śavāsana** sounds like sha-VAAH-sa-na. Pronunciation is of course influenced by a speaker's mother tongue – be it English, Hindi, Gujarati or your own native language – but trying to pronounce the words according to the spelling and diacritics is an important step towards respecting the origins of yoga.

As you advance through your yoga journey, you may wish to refine your Sanskrit pronunciation, in which case you can look online for International Alphabet of Sanskrit Transliteration (IAST) pronunciation guides and websites.* It's also worth noting that diacritics are often left out of some Western sources, particularly online, so referencing these guides can be very helpful.

For now, though, my teacher Prasad Rangnekar has kindly offered his insight into the correct pronunciation of some common Sanskrit terms, which I've listed below. This will help make your reading experience as smooth as possible, and it's something you can return to as needed:

Āsana – 'aa-sun-uh'
Āyurveda – 'aa-yur-ved-uh'
Chakra – 'chuh-kruh'
Dhāraṇā – 'dhaar-un-aah'

* The IAST was implemented by scholars in the 19th century to help individuals read ancient Indian scriptures in the most authentic way.

Dharma - 'dhur-muh'
Dhyāna - 'dhyaan-uh'
Guru - 'goo-roo'
Karma - 'kurm-uh'
Kriyā - 'kree-yaa'
Mokṣa - 'moksh-uh'
Namaskāra - 'nuhmus-kaar-uh'
Prāṇa - 'praan-uh'
Puruṣa - 'puru-sha'
Sādhanā - 'saad-hun-ah'
Samādhi - 'sam-aa-dhi'
Yama - 'yum-uh'

Part One

Why we should aim for an authentic yoga practice

Yoga has been practised in India for thousands of years, but from the 20th century onwards we've seen yoga's popularity explode in the Western world, too. Today, yoga in the Western world is considered a mainstream form of exercise (or stretching) with yoga studios and yoga influencers popping up everywhere you look.

Along with yoga's popularity, though, problems have arisen. This is because the 'yoga' that's practised in the Western world today has developed, in reality, as a warped form of traditional yoga – a version of 'modern yoga' if you will. This modern yoga has emerged as Western society has extracted certain elements from traditional yoga (bringing them into yoga spaces, wellness communities and mental health spaces), while other elements of traditional yoga have been left behind. As a result, the majority of the yoga that we see in the Western world today is completely unrecognisable from yoga as it's practised in its most traditional and authentic form.

The intentions of modern yoga teachers and practitioners in the Western world are often well-meaning, but the effects of this modern yoga can be concerning. For example, it can put unnecessary pressure on the practitioner to look or move in a certain way and it can also create a cultural divide between those who have ancestral ties to the practice and those who are unfamiliar with yoga's origins. Problems such as these arise from the disconnect between modern yoga and traditional yoga, and exploring these will be our focus in **Part 1**.

I appreciate that some of this section may be an uncomfortable read (especially if you have never considered the issues with modern yoga before), but I do encourage you to stick with it. Unpicking modern yoga and identifying its weaknesses is key in helping us understand *why* it's so important to learn about traditional yoga in its authentic form.

To help us navigate this topic, I have identified four significant points (or 'problems') for us to explore, and we'll look at each one in turn. A caveat before we begin: the scope of these topics is huge and therefore it's impossible to give anything more than an overview here, so I do invite you to explore these further yourself if you wish.

In **Part 1**, we will be looking at the following four problems of modern yoga:

Problem 1 - The emphasis on physicality in modern yoga
Problem 2 - Cultural appropriation in modern yoga
Problem 3 - Commercialisation in modern yoga
Problem 4 - The lack of diversity in modern yoga

Key terms

For clarity, I have collated some key terms that I will be using while discussing modern yoga. Please note that some of these definitions have been adapted to fit the context of my discussion of yoga.

- **Western/modern yoga** - Yoga that focuses on physical poses and doesn't include any cultural or spiritual significance.
- **Authentic/traditional yoga** - Yoga that is taught and practised while respecting and aligning with the practice's origins and traditions.
- **POC/BIPOC** - People of colour/Black, Indigenous, people of colour
- **Whitewashing** - The popularisation of yoga that erases the origins and culture of yoga while excluding BIPOC. This is done to cater mainly to white audiences, making yoga seem more acceptable or comfortable for them.

1

Problem 1: The emphasis on physicality in modern yoga

Classes structured around poses

When you attend a yoga class or participate in a yoga space today, do you feel like you've given your body or your mind a workout? I'd guess some might say both but the vast majority, if pushed to choose between the two, would probably say that yoga is mainly a workout for their body. And this is understandable given that modern yoga is typically presented as a fitness workout with classes centred around physical yoga poses.

A typical modern yoga class, for example, looks something like this: a teacher positions themselves at the front of the room, or walks around the class, as they lead students through a series of poses, sometimes offering assistance to the students by suggesting physical adjustments to help them achieve the pose correctly. The students are typically all on yoga mats and at the beginning of the class the teacher will let the students know if any further yoga props will be required to help them achieve the yoga poses. For example, the teacher may recommend yoga bricks, bolsters or straps. Usually, classes begin with a calming 5 minutes and conclude with 5–10 minutes of **Śavāsana** (a final resting pose). Success in the class is typically measured by the ability to achieve the poses, and if someone were to attend yoga classes regularly then one would assume that the person is generally physically fit and healthy.

In addition, there are numerous different 'types' of yoga classes available on the market. Timetables at yoga studios and local gyms in the Western world often display a selection of different classes, including **Haṭha**, **Yin**,

Vinyāsa Flow, **Aṣṭāṅga**, **Iyengar** and many more. And what is it about these classes that make them different from each other? You guessed it: the types of physical poses on offer. In **Yin** yoga the poses are held for 3 to 5 minutes, whereas in **Vinyāsa** yoga the poses are held for 3 to 5 breaths. The types of yoga classes available are normally defined primarily by the physical poses they teach you, with very little to no historical or cultural context given to these poses or yoga as a wider practice.

What's wrong with this focus on the physical aspects of yoga, you may ask? Well, these poses actually make up very little of what traditional yoga has to offer. Traditional yoga in its authentic form is instead a holistic practice that encompasses not only physical but also emotional, mental and spiritual elements. Typically, traditional yoga dedicates more time to these non-physical aspects (which we'll learn about in **Part 2** and **Part 3**).

Therefore, modern yoga's focus on physical poses, put simply, means that Western practitioners are participating in a fairly narrow and superficial understanding of what yoga is, while missing out on the wealth of benefits that yoga's traditional approach has to offer. Imagine yoga as a gigantic piece of embroidery with many threads – physical postures, meditation, philosophy and more, all working together. In Western yoga, often only one thread of this embroidery is explored, meaning participants are missing the opportunity to fully appreciate the depth of the practice and to see the full picture.

Is it wrong to focus solely on the physical postures of yoga?

In short, no. **Āsana** (physical postures) are indeed a fundamental aspect of yoga, so there's nothing inherently wrong with practising them alone.

However, it's important to reflect on your reasons for practising these postures. Are you simply treating yoga as a form of physical exercise, such as going to the gym, with a focus solely on increased flexibility and strength? Or do you view the physical poses as just one part of a broader yoga practice, understanding and respecting its wider history and culture?

→

You see, issues can arise when yoga poses are pursued purely for physical benefits. I mention this not to discourage anyone from exploring yoga, but to stress the significance of understanding your intentions when entering yoga spaces, so that we can avoid diluting the integrity of the practice.

If you're primarily drawn to yoga poses for their physical effects, I can relate to that motivation. Initially, I was attracted to yoga poses because I hoped they would help alleviate discomfort from my injury and loosen my muscles. But if you're only interested in the physical aspects of yoga, you might consider referring to your practice as '**yoga āsana**' ('yoga poses') rather than simply 'yoga'. This would help avoid you contributing to any misunderstandings surrounding yoga and what the practice means.

Ideally, when practising yoga poses, we would all have an understanding and respect for yoga's history, roots and complexities to add context to our physical practice, and reading this book is a great start. I'll be sharing practical ways to expand your engagement with yoga (beyond the physical) throughout, with a particular focus on this in **Part 3**.

I'll leave you with the wisdom of Swami Jnaneshvara Bharati, who said that it's false to think 'yoga is a physical system with a spiritual component' and instead it is true to think 'yoga is a spiritual system with a physical component.' In an ideal world, every practitioner of yoga should be aiming to embody this approach.

Pressure to push yourself too far

Imagine you or I, as complete beginners, searching for 'yoga' on social media platforms now. I guarantee that the images and videos that pop up will include super-flexible people performing intense yoga poses, such as backbends or splits. A big concern with modern yoga's presentation of 'yoga as movement' lies in the pressure this creates for practitioners, especially beginners, to pursue postures that are too physically advanced. Attempting these advanced poses can lead to feelings of inadequacy and even danger at times if a practitioner pushes themself too far. Let's explore both of these ideas further.

Feelings of inadequacy

Walking into my first modern yoga class in my early twenties, I remember looking around and feeling quite intimidated. Several thoughts ran through my head, such as 'Do I have the flexibility that yoga requires?' and 'What if my body can't bend like everyone else's here?' I know that I'm certainly not alone in having experienced these insecurities on entering a class, and when we consider how yoga in the Western world is presented it's really not surprising.

The set-up of a modern yoga class today, as we've discussed, is such that the focus is on achieving poses and keeping up with the class. Even if this pressure is not facilitated by the teacher or other practitioners, the whole environment is so centred around physical poses that it is easy for feelings of inadequacy, doubt or frustration to creep in if you struggle to keep up with the pace of the class or to perform the poses 'correctly'. It's therefore common practice in class for seasoned practitioners to confidently line themselves up at the front to showcase their ability to move and flex, while beginners often place themselves at the back for fear of publicly falling behind or lacking flexibility.

Even accepting modifications in class from a teacher or needing to use a yoga prop to help you reach a certain pose can make you feel like you're behind. However, not accepting these modifications and adjustments (more on p. 172) can cause you to struggle, risking injury or discomfort, which leads us nicely on to the next point...

Dangerous practices leading to injury

Injury is common in modern yoga and, if we think about it, it's not surprising. Pressure in class can lead practitioners to be more focused on keeping pace rather than staying attuned to their own bodies, which means we can put ourselves in danger of pushing ourselves beyond our physical boundaries.

The presentation of advanced poses, both online and in class, can also contribute to competitive behaviour in the yoga world, which yoga teachers themselves are not immune to. In 2019, the *Daily Telegraph* shed light on this concerning trend as it reported that '[yoga] instructors are falling victim to more injuries because they are rushing into attempting challenging poses that will look good on social media'.

It also found that 'Instagram is fuelling [a] rise in injuries amongst yoga teachers who want [the] perfect social media post.' Aspirational poses in modern yoga can therefore not only hurt our self-esteem but also our bodies if we fall victim to pushing ourselves too hard to reach 'social media standards'.

I have a confession here: I was one of those individuals myself. Back in 2019, I began attempting handstands at home with very little guidance and hardly any experience. I soon made it my goal to be able to hold a handstand, or even a forearm stand, for more than five seconds without the assistance of the wall or a teacher. Although I did seek out the help of a teacher eventually, the constant push on myself to achieve this pose, which I thought would prove my worth in the yoga world, made me forget to listen to my body. I lost sight of the fact that I'm not completely able-bodied (as discussed on p. 15), which I need to consider when attempting certain postures. A few months into my challenge I caused further injury to my ongoing back condition and was completely bed-bound for three weeks. I had pushed my body so hard that I ended up tearing a muscle around my already fractured spine.

I may not have wanted to admit it at the time, but the truth is that I only set out on my handstand journey because of what I was seeing on my social media feed: experienced yoga teachers performing inversions and fancy poses. The constant exposure to this narrative made me put myself at risk, but my injury did help me see clearly that inversions weren't the be-all and end-all of my, or anyone else's, yoga practice, especially if it meant causing harm to myself. It can be so easy to overlook your own mental and physical state, though, when you get caught up in comparison. Here we can see exactly how modern yoga - without any authentic knowledge from traditional yoga grounding us - can be harmful to beginners today. (Don't worry, though, because I'll be showing you how we can practise the physical aspects of yoga safely and comfortably later, in **Part 3**).

Yoga and comparison

If you get caught on the train of comparison within modern yoga, here are two things to remember:

1. Some people are naturally more flexible.
2. Some people have athletic backgrounds - being dancers, swimmers, gymnasts etc. - that you may not necessarily know about.

In other words, some people have a physical head-start in terms of 'achieving' the physical poses and this isn't necessarily always a result of a dedicated yoga practice. This isn't to invalidate these people, it's just a reminder for anyone who is reading this and may not feel 'good enough' while practising the physical aspects of yoga.

The hyper-sexualisation of yoga

As we've mentioned, searching for 'yoga' on social media today delivers content of (mainly) women performing advanced and aspirational physical yoga poses. One element we haven't touched on yet, though, is the way that so much of this yoga content online is highly sexualised. Take TikTok, for example. This platform can often be used for educational purposes and does a great job at it! However, when searching for yoga on this platform it falls short when it comes to authentic yoga representation.

The top TikTok searches for yoga (at the time of writing) contain accounts using yoga to promote products or services unrelated to the practice and of a sexual nature. These videos feature practitioners in sexually suggestive poses and often dressed in minimal clothing, with legs spread apart or contorted in ways that emphasise certain private body parts. This is the same with Instagram, where some of the top yoga accounts have grown sizeable followings by featuring yoga practitioners in highly unattainable and highly sexualised postures. We even see studios or brands using sexualised imagery in their advertising, and creators using suggestive captions to promote their own yoga businesses. (If you're not sure what I'm talking about then feel free to take a moment now to explore 'yoga' on social media and see what you discover.)

So, what's the problem with this? Well, the hyper-sexualisation of yoga often leads to the objectification of yoga practitioners, especially women. I can't count how many times I have told a man that I'm a yoga teacher, only for their response to be, 'So you must be *really* flexible ;)'. This makes me want to walk away from them every time! The hyper-sexualisation of yoga leaves us with damaging stereotypes and further draws attention to the Physical Body in yoga which, as we discussed, means our attention is fixated on one tiny part of what yoga has to offer. Also, the hyper-sexualisation of yoga for *external* validation fundamentally feels disrespectful and wrong, when considering that the true meaning of yoga is about our *internal* work and self-reflection (as we'll explore in **Part 2** and **Part 3**).

A moment of introspection

You may now be able to notice how focussing too much on physical postures in yoga can make it difficult for some people to start practicing. Take a moment to think about these questions:

- Have you ever felt pressured to compare yourself to others in your yoga class or environment?
- Has the way yoga is often sexualised ever made you hesitant to try it?
- Are there other ways you can think of where the focus on the physical side of yoga might discourage people from beginning?

2

Problem 2: Cultural appropriation in modern yoga

Cultural appropriation is the second problem we'll explore when identifying the weaknesses of modern yoga. It's interesting because while the cultural appropriation of yoga has become a popular topic in the Western world over recent years, there's still such a lack of understanding about what this actually means and how it can manifest itself in modern yoga today. Let's look at this now.

Q. What is cultural appropriation?

A. 'Cultural appropriation takes place when members of a majority group adopt cultural elements of a minority group in an exploitative, disrespectful, or stereotypical way.' – Britannica

To demonstrate how this can show up in real life, let me share a broad example. In a popular TV show from the 1990s, there was a scene in which a statue of Lord Ganesha (a Hindu deity) was placed on a table in one of the character's apartments. During the scene, the actor put their legs on the table, kicking the idol off. I remember being in shock when I first saw this. As a Hindu, we're taught to treat these deities with the utmost respect. Hindu idols should always be placed on an altar or platform and treated with reverence, exactly how you would treat a holy place of worship. Placing these deities on the floor or using them carelessly as a superficial decoration (or as a prop in a TV show in this instance) is disrespectful and can be considered a form of cultural appropriation.

Q. What is cultural appropriation in yoga?

A. When we relate cultural appropriation directly to yoga, we are referring to the act of using traditional yogic practices, techniques, terminology and symbols in the Western world with little to no acknowledgement (or even understanding) of their cultural significance in Indian culture. The chosen 'popular' elements taken from traditional yoga are then distorted and served up in the Western world to a predominantly white audience, forming part of what we recognise today as modern yoga. Let's look at some specific ways this can play out...

The use of yogic terms and symbols as trends

The use of certain terms and symbols in modern yoga is a clear example of cultural appropriation within the practice. To demonstrate this, we'll now explore two terms that hold deep significance in Hinduism and Indian culture that are commonly misused or misunderstood in the context of modern yoga (whether this be in the practice itself or in the marketing and branding surrounding the practice). These are: **namaste** and **mantras**.

Namaste

Namaste (pronounced 'nuh-muh-stey') is a Sanskrit term that is commonly used as a way of closing a yoga class in the Western world. It is also one of the words that is most commonly associated with the modern yoga world more generally. But increasingly its use in yoga has been up for debate with some modern yoga teachers and practitioners now choosing to leave it out of their practice completely. Let's explore why.

According to the **Vedas** (the ancient Hindu texts we'll explore on p. 75), **namaste** can be used either as a salutation to divinity or as a means of greeting, and showing respect and gratitude, to others and to deities. **Namaste** means 'I offer my respect to you' or 'the divine in me acknowledges the divine in you'. Traditionally, **namaste** is usually practised while also adopting a specific hand gesture called ***añjali mudrā***, which involves pressing your palms together at the heart centre. From understanding the meaning behind **namaste**, we can therefore see that using this term to end a yoga class does make sense to some degree.

However, the use of **namaste** has become more problematic in recent times since the term has become 'trendy' and we've seen it increasingly used as an 'accessory' to yoga. You may have seen brands creating clothing or other merchandise with slogans to exploit the term, such as 'Namastay in bed' or 'Namaste, Bitches'. Using the word in this way completely strips it of its meaning and cultural significance, and therefore this can be seen as cultural appropriation. It is also deemed hugely disrespectful to some of the Indian population who class **namaste** as a sacred expression.

Should we therefore stop using **namaste** completely, you may be wondering? I personally have stopped using it during my practice due to the extent of its appropriation. For example, I now prefer to use alternative ways of closing my class, such as a simple 'thank you' or another way of expressing gratitude. However, when considering if you would like to use **namaste** as part of your practice, the key thing for you to consider is your intention behind using the term. I suggest you ask yourself: 'Am I being mindful and respectful of **namaste**'s true meaning? Does using the term feel authentic to me?' Your answers to these questions will help you understand what the right decision is for you.

Mantras

Mantras are sacred sounds or phrases thought to generate a spiritual energy field around us, aiding our connection to something greater than ourselves (such as the divine). The word **mantra** is a Sanskrit term that means 'mind tool' or 'mind instrument', so you can think of **mantras** as tools that can transform our mental and spiritual well-being. The more we repeat a **mantra** (either out loud or silently), the more potent its effect is believed to be, making repetition key for enhancing its power. **Mantras** can have different purposes, such as protection, healing, blessings and more. Common examples of **mantras** are the sound '**om**' (or 'aum') or '**Oṃ Namaḥ Śivāya**' (which means 'I bow down to Shiva'), and these **mantras** are often used during meditation to focus the mind.

Traditionally, **mantras** were transmitted from guru* to student within specific lineages to ensure that their profound significance and proper usage were preserved. However, in modern yoga, it's common to see

* A **guru** is a spiritual mentor or guide.

'**mantras**' introduced without this spiritual context, which dilutes their meaning and leads to a lack of appreciation for them. For example, a teacher might casually incorporate '**Oṃ Namaḥ Śivāya**' without any explanation of its meaning or its connection to the deity Lord Shiva. Or we often see '**mantras**' used interchangeably with affirmations. This means the understanding of true **mantras** can be reduced to just positive statements, such as 'I am stronger than I know.' Although I am not against the use of affirmations, **mantras** are much more than an uplifting phrase to increase positivity. This superficial use of '**mantras**' within modern yoga – without an understanding of their cultural and spiritual roots – can be viewed as cultural appropriation.

To respect the sacredness of **mantras** and honour the tradition of yoga, **mantras** need to be taught by a teacher who is well-versed in yogic traditions and culture. This ensures that **mantras** are taught and practised with the reverence and context they deserve.

A note on om

Om is a **mantra** that consists of three sounds: A-U-M. Within Hinduism, it signifies the source of creation and consciousness. Traditionally, **om** is used during yogic practices, such as meditation, and it's also used at the beginning and/or end of prayers during sacred Hindu ceremonies.

Om is probably the most popular **mantra** used in modern yoga. It is commonly reduced to a chant at the end of a yoga class, without any explanation. When a meaning is given, it's often the oversimplification that **om** represents the sound of the universe.

Unfortunately, in broader Western contexts, the significance of **om** is frequently watered down, used more for its visual appeal or marketing value than for its profound spiritual meaning. It's disheartening to see **om** become a trendy fashion statement, appearing on jewellery and tattoos, even in inappropriate places such as the feet. Additionally, using **om** as a design on yoga mats is considered cultural appropriation, as sacred symbols should be placed respectfully on altars or platforms and treated with utmost reverence.

→

While **om** holds deep significance in Hinduism and Buddhism, its usage in Western wellness settings often lacks authenticity, with little consideration for its spiritual origins. Instead, it's used as a superficial aesthetic or to add an exotic flair to yoga classes.

As with **mantras** and **namaste**, using **om** with an understanding of its cultural and spiritual significance is very important in preserving the roots of yoga.

Practising yoga with animals and alcohol

Hands up if you've ever heard of yoga classes that involve puppies, goats, intense heat, paddle boards ... or even wine(!)? These days, the term 'yoga' can be added on to anything and sold as 'yoga', and these types of novelty classes have become very popular. But why are they a problem?

Well, first, let's be clear – these novelty classes are not *really* yoga. They're simply gimmicks to make money. Practising yoga with any form of distraction present (whether that be loud, inappropriate music, animals or wine) detracts from the internal stillness that yoga in its truest form encourages us to cultivate (and we'll explore this more in **Part 3**). For example, how much inner peace can one truly achieve while wobbling around on a paddle board for 'Paddle Board Yoga'? (I think this would be a challenge for most!) And while it may seem cute to have puppies cuddling up to you during a 'Puppy Yoga' class, the animals will of course be a distraction from you cultivating your inner self-awareness, not to mention raising ethical concerns about animal welfare. A recent article in the *Guardian* highlighted young puppies being unfairly treated as working animals and reportedly being deprived of water to avoid them urinating during classes.

And as for yoga with alcohol? This goes against yogic philosophy completely as the principles of traditional yoga that we'll be exploring – self-discipline, moderation and awareness – are all at odds with alcohol consumption.

Despite what one might see in 'trendy' Western yoga scenes, yoga isn't supposed to be a 'fun' or an 'entertaining' practice. Sure, you can have fun while practising, but prioritising fun over mindfulness and other key yogic principles hugely misses the mark. Imagine 'Rowing with Puppies' or 'Beer and HIIT' classes – sounds a bit odd, doesn't it? That's exactly how these yoga fads sound to those who are from the source culture of yoga, or even for those who aren't but have been practising yoga for a while!

The introduction of these novelty yoga classes, which selectively adopt elements of yoga while disregarding its rich cultural heritage, is another example of how the practice is culturally appropriated in the West. Packaging up yoga as 'entertainment' in this way is a version of yoga that strays far from yoga's Indian origins.

Naked yoga

There has been controversy surrounding another type of 'yoga' that has been made available in recent times – naked yoga.

Can we practise yoga without our clothes on? Well, that's entirely up to you and what you're comfortable with in your own space at home. But while what you choose to wear (or not wear) during your private yoga practice is your personal decision, classes like 'Naked Yoga' can raise some concerns. In these classes, the focus tends to be solely on nudity, often sidelining the cultural aspects of yoga. This can lead to questions about the true intention behind these classes – are they about genuine yoga practice or simply for profit and shock factor?

Cultural appropriation vs cultural appreciation

Hopefully you should now have a sense of how to spot cultural appropriation within modern yoga and we'll be learning throughout **Part 2** and **Part 3** how to turn any cultural appropriation into cultural appreciation. By 'cultural appreciation' I mean when we recognise and respect the traditions of yoga. To help you understand this, I've summarised on the following page some of the main points we've discussed so far in **Part 1** and separated them out into cultural appropriation vs cultural appreciation.

Cultural appropriation in yoga	Cultural appreciation in yoga
Using yoga purely as a fitness or workout regime while disregarding the spirituality and cultural context of yoga.	Benefitting from the physical poses in yoga to help with movement, but also acknowledging and incorporating other aspects of yoga, such as **prāṇāyāma** (breath control), **mudrā** (gestures), **dhyāna** (meditation) and **kriyās** (cleansing practices). We'll be exploring these further in **Part 3**.
Taking any of the cultural elements of yoga and monetising or using them for personal gain. For example, creating or wearing activewear with yogic terms such as **namaste** plastered on them with an inappropriate context, such as 'Namastay, Bitches'.	Taking cultural elements of yoga and incorporating them into your practice. For example, using the Sanskrit language to reference the physical poses in yoga, and having an understanding of the yogic texts and scriptures (as we'll discuss in **Part 2**) to help deepen your practice.
Classes such as 'Puppy Yoga', 'Goat Yoga', 'Beer Yoga', 'Wine Yoga', 'Drunk Yoga', 'Hot Yoga', 'Paddle Board Yoga', 'Naked Yoga' or classes with loud or inappropriate music.	Learning yoga by attending classes led by teachers who practise cultural appreciation themselves in the most respectful and authentic way.

A moment of introspection

To help you embrace cultural appreciation in your yoga journey, I invite you to take stock by considering the following:

1. Can you think of any ways that cultural appropriation might show up in your current practice?
2. What is one simple step you can take to include more cultural appreciation in your current practice?

3

Problem 3: Commercialisation in modern yoga

As yoga has grown in the Western world, so too has the commercialisation surrounding it as brands and studios have seized the opportunity to profit from yoga's popularity. But when yoga is commercialised in this way, two main problems emerge: 1) a financial barrier to entry and 2) modern yoga becomes increasingly distant from its traditional roots. Let's explore these further.

The cost of practising yoga

Yoga can be an incredibly fulfilling and enriching practice but, in the Western world, it can also be quite expensive.

Search for a yoga retreat today and you'll find that each one promises serenity and immersion from the world in a blissful setting. But each one also comes with a price tag that might give your wallet a bit of a workout! Whether you're paying for individual classes, purchasing a monthly studio membership, attending one-off courses or going to festivals and workshops, the costs of yoga in the Western world can quickly add up. Although some gyms or studios may offer introductory pricing or drop-in rates, the majority of workshops and classes today demand high fees. This financial investment is great for the business or studio looking to make profit, but it can create a significant barrier for many practitioners who wish to access yoga.

Yoga teacher training, in particular, requires a significant investment by aspiring teachers. The cost of the learning materials required, the course itself and any potential travel expenses (if you wish to train abroad) can be daunting.

So, what's the deal with the cost of practising yoga in the Western world? The offerings available do provide people with access to yoga, which is great, but it's clear that money is what is prioritised*. Simply put: companies are charging so much for access to yoga because they can. The demand is there. In the Western world, yoga has been turned into a product to sell, and a popular one at that.

This means yoga often comes with hefty price tags, making studio classes and retreats inaccessible for many. This, in turn, means modern yoga has morphed into an exclusive pastime. Businesses, of course, do need to make money, but charging so much for classes and access has ultimately infused a level of commodification into yoga that distances modern yoga far from traditional yoga, where the core value is of inclusivity for all. This loss – and separation between the two forms of yoga – is not something to be overlooked lightly.

The cost of clothing and equipment

Yoga's popularity in modern times has brought about a newfound emphasis on yoga clothing and equipment in the West. However, the trend of owning expensive leggings or mats can sometimes send the wrong message, suggesting that specific attire and kit are essential for practising yoga.

This focus on 'stuff' has led to the marketing of yoga clothing and equipment at prices that may not be accessible for everyone, especially those on a budget. If you're new to yoga and browse social media, you might notice practitioners wearing luxury yoga wear from big brands. While there's nothing inherently wrong with wearing branded clothing to practise yoga, there is something wrong when yoga becomes so centred around specific brands that people feel they can't join in if they don't own or can't afford certain items. Labelling

* I'm mainly talking about my experience with yoga studios in big Western cities like London and New York that can charge upwards of £20 for one class. Local yoga classes, in village halls for example, are often more affordable but seem to be sadly disappearing in areas where brands are taking over.

leggings as 'yoga pants' allows companies to attach a high price tag to them, when really there is nothing yogic about those pants! The overall effect of this is that it makes yoga seem very exclusive. (And if this is how yoga is promoted, it's no wonder beginners feel intimidated when approaching the practice!)

Equally, the focus on expensive equipment, like yoga mats, has become prominent in the Western world. With a vast selection of mats differing in quality, design and material, it's easy to get lost in the sea of options. Some equipment such as yoga wheels or headstand props can be helpful, but they can disingenuously be marketed as essential for the practice, creating a perception that owning expensive items is necessary to participate.

As well as causing an accessibility issue, this commercialisation has raised concerns surrounding inclusivity, particularly for marginalised groups. For instance, certain prominent activewear brands have faced criticism for failing to offer inclusive sizing options, especially for plus-size women, while also pricing their products at unreasonably high levels. Despite bragging about excellent fits, innovative design features and great quality, some of these well-known brands have been notorious for perpetuating body shaming. This again only serves to associate modern yoga with values that are completely at odds with traditional yoga's core values of inclusivity.

By holding these brands accountable and advocating for more inclusive policies, we can work towards creating a more equitable and accessible space for all practitioners today.

So, what do I really need in order to practise yoga?

Contrary to what you might think, you don't *need* anything but yourself to practise yoga. I'll repeat this again: to practise yoga you do not need anything at all apart from yourself. A mat, a block, a bolster, yoga leggings, a membership to a top studio or any other additions you can think of are all *optional* (i.e. not essential!) to your practice. I talk more about props later on p. 173, but here's my take on the following:

- **Clothing** - It isn't a must to be able to purchase expensive clothing from top brands. *Wearing clothing that makes you feel good in your practice* is.
- **Equipment** - High-end equipment is not crucial to your practice. *Being able to make use of what is around you, such as books or pillows instead of blocks and bolsters,* is.
- **Yoga mats** - These don't play a major role in your practice. *Your mind and body* do.

Being a 'good' yoga teacher or practitioner doesn't require high-end clothing or equipment despite what is depicted through mainstream yoga. In fact, this tendency to centre material items in Western yoga spaces can take the focus away from the real reason why you might be showing up for class in the first place.

Let's just say, you need less than you think to build a regular practice. An open mind and a spirit for learning and growing is enough to get you started on your yogic path, despite what you may be being sold.

4

Problem 4: The lack of diversity in modern yoga

Yoga in its genuine, traditional form (as we'll explore in **Part 3**) is founded on core principles that emphasise accessibility, inclusivity and respect for all living beings. Yoga carries many benefits for practitioners on a mental, physical and emotional level that could benefit everyone, yet we rarely see yoga in the Western world being made accessible to all. This is because many well-intentioned people, including myself, have *unintentionally* created modern yoga spaces that did not feel inclusive for everyone. The lack of diversity is therefore the final problem that we will address when it comes to yoga in the modern Western world.

This is an important topic to shed light on because we all share the responsibility of working to make yoga accessible to everyone. It is our collective responsibility to create safe and inviting yoga environments where everyone is appreciated and valued. The first step in rectifying this and taking steps towards creating safe and inclusive yoga spaces (which are more aligned with traditional yoga's values) is for us to understand the situation, so that's what we'll look more closely at now.

Key terms

Some of the main themes we'll be working through are listed below, so let's get clear on what these terms mean:

- **Accessibility** - Information, practices or activities that are easy to approach and usable for EVERYONE.
- **Inclusivity** - Maximising diversity regardless of social status or orientation and making sure everyone has equal access to opportunities and resources.

→

- **Diversity** – Promoting, involving and embracing people of all social groups and identities.
- **Marginalised communities** – Groups of people who encounter societal disadvantages and are often excluded from mainstream life due to systemic inequalities, discrimination and limited access to resources and opportunities.

Yoga and marginalised communities

Let's begin by seeing how certain marginalised communities are often left out of modern yoga. Before we dive in, a quick disclaimer: I want to acknowledge that I am continually learning every day and I do not claim to be an expert in social justice. I cannot speak for the experiences of everyone and please know that your specific experience is valid even if it is not detailed here. What I can do is present an account here of what I have experienced and witnessed myself on my own journey with modern yoga. I have also shared the voices of others from marginalised communities as they reflect on their own relationship with yoga on p. 62. I remain open to expanding my understanding.

Socio-economic status

Yoga in the Western world is often marketed as a high-end form of fitness with expensively priced classes. This can make yoga less accessible to individuals from lower-income backgrounds who may struggle to afford these classes. When we talk about accessibility in yoga, we're talking about financial access, too.

Race and ethnicity

In the context of yoga, there are clear racial biases (and we will explore this more deeply on p. 58). Although these biases may not be apparent to white practitioners, the Western yoga community does often appear to favour white individuals. This is apparent when we see predominantly white teachers employed in wellness spaces or when predominantly white practitioners are chosen to represent yoga brands through advertising. Whether the biases that BIPOC encounter in yoga are as a result of conscious or unconscious discrimination, they certainly exist. This creates a sense of exclusion for anyone from a diverse racial background and makes them feel like they don't truly belong in the modern yoga space.

Sexual orientation

There have also been instances where LGBTQIA+ individuals have faced challenges in finding inclusive spaces that cater to their needs. For example, yoga marketing has very often excluded LGBTQIA+ individuals from their campaigns and this lack of representation can make people from the community feel invisible. Being asked inappropriate questions or being treated differently within the yoga space can also leave LGBTQIA+ individuals feeling unwelcome, unsafe or unsupported. This reinforces the idea that yoga is only for a specific demographic.

Body shape or size

Western yoga often glorifies slender bodies and the ability to carry out advanced poses, as we discussed on p. 37. The 'ideal' yoga body type is often portrayed in yoga marketing and on social media as slim and flexible, and other body types are rarely featured. This invalidates anyone who does not fit this stereotypical 'ideal' because if you don't see anyone who resembles yourself in the practice, or in the media surrounding the practice, you'll often be less inclined to participate.

Additionally, modern yoga can exclude individuals if the yoga clothing and props are designed only to fit standard body sizes, which is often the case. It can be challenging for people with larger bodies to find suitable attire or equipment for their practice, which does not make them feel welcome in the space.

Disabilities

As modern yoga places a great emphasis on being super-flexible and able to achieve physical yoga poses, discrimination against people who have disabilities (i.e. ableism) is prevalent in yoga. The common excuse of 'I'm not flexible enough' when asked why someone doesn't practise yoga only highlights this issue. Traditional yoga is highly accessible for people with disabilities, so the fact that modern yoga presents as highly inaccessible to the wider disabled community is cause for concern. People with mental disabilities also often face discrimination in modern yoga spaces due to a lack of representation and inadequate support for their needs.

Non-vegans

A misconception that surrounds modern yoga is that you must adhere to a strict diet, often one that complies with the yogic principle of **ahiṃsā** (non-harm). This has been fixated on by some within the modern yoga community and, as a result, there have been many instances where people have expressed their concerns about feeling pressure to adopt veganism within yoga communities.

With veganism being a concept that has been popularised by Western societies, modern yoga practitioners have often overlooked the true historical context of yoga in relation to veganism, because in traditional yoga teachings there is no explicit claim of a vegan lifestyle. In fact, ancient yogis often incorporated animal products into their diets, although sourced ethically.

The idea that being vegan is the only way to practise **ahiṃsā**, or any part of yoga, reinforces exclusion in yoga for those unable to adhere to a vegan lifestyle due to accessibility or health constraints. I've received many messages from beginners in my online community thanking me for talking about veganism and yoga. One message that really stood out to me was from someone who has autism and sensory issues, which limits the food they can eat. They thought yogic living wasn't an option for them because meat and dairy are an essential part of their limited diet. But that's simply not the case. I touch on the requirements of a yogic diet in more detail on p. 140.

Age

Yoga classes and spaces can also be intimidating for older adults as the practice of modern yoga is usually youth-oriented. The focus on physical poses, and the pose hierarchy that places advanced yoga postures at the top, suggests that yoga is solely for those who are young and fit. This can make older adults feel discouraged to practise, believing that yoga is not suitable for them. Again, there are very few appearances of older adults when it comes to mainstream yoga marketing.

Caste

Exploring the intricate nature of caste warrants more space than we have here, but I feel it's crucial to touch on the issue, especially given its relevance to my work as a yoga instructor.

The caste system (referred to as **varna** in Sanskrit) is a longstanding social hierarchy in India dating back to the Vedic age. It categorises people into four castes based on their birth, occupation and social status. Traditionally, the **varnas** included Kshatriyas (warriors and rulers), Brahmins (priests and scholars), Vaishyas (farmers, traders and merchants) and Shudras (labourers and servants) and each was associated with specific roles and responsibilities. The concept of caste existed in ancient India, but it was reinforced under British colonial rule. It was also during this time that the caste system was restructured to exploit people of lower castes.

The barriers caused by the caste system, whether intentional or systemic, can still pose an accessibility issue for practitioners in the modern day. For example, a person from a lower-class background may face social discrimination that makes it difficult for them to access certain yoga spaces or teachings.

For anyone seeking to dive deeper into the subject of yoga's accessibility, understanding the caste system and its historical implications is important to create safe and inclusive yoga environments.

All in all, I think that what we've just discussed can be summed up rather nicely by the findings of a 2019 study that analysed the coverage of yoga and accessibility within mainstream yoga media. The report found: 'limited visual representations of men, older adults, people of colour, and people of larger body size, and that these representations have become increasingly narrow over the past four decades, potentially discouraging people from trying yoga despite its health benefits.' At the heart of traditional yoga is a practice that many marginalised individuals could greatly benefit from, but from which they often feel excluded.

This is unfortunate as the practice of yoga has several health benefits, such as stress reduction and managing symptoms of anxiety and depression (which we will talk about later), so yoga can be a great tool for coping with life's hurdles when practised by individuals who experience social inequalities. I have already mentioned some of my physical and mental health conditions, and I am fortunate enough to have access to the care I need. However, this isn't always the case for everyone. Think about those who have reduced access to healthcare. Could yoga act as an alternative means of assisting your mental health and give you tools to cope? One hundred per cent yes! Many BIPOC individuals face obstacles to gaining access to mental health care and therefore inclusive yoga is essential for our well-being. However, the barriers that marginalised communities are faced with when it comes to accessing yoga sometimes prevent the practice from reaching those people.

Accessibility in yoga as we know it today is often overlooked. However, traditional yoga strives to be inclusive and doesn't discriminate against anyone regardless of background, status, ability or body type. Yoga in its most authentic form is highly adaptable and can always be modified to serve everyone's needs and purposes. When we use yoga in this traditional way, we make it available to anyone who wishes to seek it. This insight only serves to highlight more clearly the problems with accessibility and modern yoga today.

Yoga and racism

People's opinions of what they deem to be the most problematic element of accessibility in modern yoga vary widely. My own most challenging and distressing experiences have been around feeling excluded from yoga in the Western world because of the colour of my skin. So, I'd like to take some time here to highlight the experience of the BIPOC community's exclusion from modern yoga.

Q. 'I'm a white woman who has practised yoga for 20 years. I have never witnessed racism in yoga. Is this really a problem?' – Anonymous social media user

A. That's understandable and I hear this a lot. That's exactly why it's so important to have these conversations and to raise awareness. These discussions might cause some discomfort, but racism does exist in modern yoga. Racism doesn't always have to be as direct as you may think and, quite often, it isn't visible to those who aren't affected by it. If you have had no personal experience of racial discrimination in yoga, then you might struggle to relate to the exclusion felt by BIPOC. But it's important to listen to other voices and learn.

Unfortunately, systemic racism manifests in yoga communities in many ways. As I heard a teacher once say: 'Our communities are the reflection of our society, therefore racism and oppression are going to be reflected in our yoga and wellness spaces.' Systemic racism doesn't always equate to hate crimes, racial slurs or actions. It is a practice that is subtly but deeply embedded in our society and results in harmful or unfair treatment of others based on race. Let's look at different ways this can show up in the modern yoga community now.

Racial bias and tokenism

We have touched on this a few times now, but racial bias (in the context of our discussion) means that spiritual and well-being spaces are predominantly reserved for white bodies. Many wellness spaces and organisations don't prioritise offering a diverse range of cultural services that resonate with different communities. For instance, lots of yoga studios mainly have classes led by white instructors, and we often see mostly white people in yoga marketing. This trend is also seen on social media platforms like YouTube, where the top results for yoga classes typically feature white individuals.

Sometimes, in instances where people of colour are seen in yoga spaces, they are tokenised or expected to represent their entire race or ethnicity. This can lead to feelings of pressure to keep up with stereotypes or to continually educate others about issues related to race and identity. When there is no intention or effort to address these gaps, these spaces feel inaccessible for teachers and practitioners from marginalised backgrounds.

My experience of tokenism

During the height of the pandemic in 2020, the Black Lives Matter movement began, and social media was flooded with black boxes as a show of solidarity. Along with this came an influx of yoga and wellness brands switching up their marketing to represent more of the BIPOC community, especially Black and Brown people. However, it became evident that some of these changes were made insincerely and were a response to the outrage from the BIPOC community during the movement. This representation was undone after just a few months and the connotation of those little black squares was soon forgotten.

It was around this time that a well-established brand asked me to become a brand ambassador for them, and I happily accepted. After accepting the offer, I once again caught sight of the lack of representation of native teachers in their branding. I wrote to the brand expressing my concerns, and initially the CEO responded sympathetically and seemed supportive. But as time went by, nothing changed. I wrote to them again, quite firmly this time, and told them I was no longer willing to represent their brand if changes weren't made. However, this time round they seemed less considerate and didn't acknowledge my concerns. So, I stood by my decision and left. For me, it was unacceptable that they profit from our heritage and culture without acknowledging or representing the people from whom it came.

Unfortunately, this was not a one-off incident. I have had many more experiences like this and soon grew tired of constantly having to ask to be seen and heard. It became clear to me that for too long, people like me have had to fight for recognition in yoga spaces.

Yoga teachers from the BIPOC community

In many yoga spaces, festivals and events it's common to see a majority of white practitioners, with only a few Black or Brown individuals present. This lack of diversity can make it difficult for BIPOC individuals to feel like they belong and can discourage them from considering teaching yoga themselves. I've had numerous aspiring teachers from the BIPOC community approach me during workshops or festivals, sharing their worries about imposter syndrome when it comes to teaching yoga because of this lack of representation. It perpetuates assumptions about who is deemed capable of teaching yoga, often resulting in the exclusion of BIPOC teachers during the hiring process.

People often speak about how underpaid yoga teachers are in the wellness industry generally, but there's not much discussion of the additional challenges faced by teachers of colour. The lack of representation affects the livelihood of teachers of colour, because it's even more challenging for them to secure jobs in the first place and sustain themselves solely through teaching yoga. As I write this, I still find myself needing a full-time job to support my yoga career. When I have approached studios, I've been turned away on multiple occasions for not having enough experience even though I have more than enough. The reality remains that I am an Indian teacher, and it's a rarity to see Indian teachers in the landscape of modern yoga.

To give you a different perspective I interviewed Tejal Patel (@tejalyoga) and Vikramjeet Singh (@wanderingmat) about their experiences of being yoga teachers of Indian heritage.

> *In India I studied Haṭha style from the Sivananda lineage. Upon returning to the US, I had 500 training hours, but studios in the West valued different styles, like vinyasa. They even suggested I gain more experience, despite my extensive training. I thought that if going to India to get training isn't enough, what is it that you actually are looking for? And that's when I started to realise that something was horribly wrong!... I think I went in thinking that everyone was well-intentioned, so they had their own business reasons for what they were saying, and I didn't want to discredit them* [by addressing the issue]. *However, the disconnect I felt between everyone else in the studio and me, and the lack of diversity I saw around me made me realize 'OK there might be something sticky here...'*
>
> – Tejal Patel, yoga teacher, writer and podcaster

> *Several years ago, I was sitting in a restaurant with a friend and sharing with her some of my insecurities about teaching yoga. At the time I was a successful teacher of over a decade, teaching 40 to 60 classes a week. My classes were full and sought after, and I always had great feedback on my teaching, yet I felt I was at a standstill*

in my career. I remember it was the weekend of the annual Yoga Conference in Toronto, and I was sharing with her that I felt a sense of sadness that I had never been asked to teach at the conference. On some level it had me question my worth as a teacher, I felt imposter syndrome, and like I didn't 'fit in' with the other teachers who were being showcased. When she probed deeper about why specifically I felt that way, I shared that despite having deep knowledge about philosophy and a well-established āsana practice, it amounted to nothing. Yoga in the West had a certain image and being a POC, I did not fit that image, and subsequently felt alienated from anything remotely mainstream or main stage. The deeper issue here is that there was (and to some extent still is) such an imbalance of authority and representation that most teachers of colour would just accept this as the norm and never question it.

My friend was in shock that I, an Indian Yoga teacher, who grew up learning the Bhagavad Gita, *chanting, and being immersed in yogic culture from a young age felt imposter syndrome next to a group of people who weren't even from my culture. But I didn't even see it. That's how insidious this was. There was such little Indian representation within mainstream yoga, and the majority of teachers being promoted and given an opportunity in the limelight were the ones who were more 'marketable'. Thankfully I have never had an overt experience of being excluded in yoga spaces, but this subtle exclusion, which had me question my worth and legitimacy as a teacher – which I think is something many South Asian teachers have felt – was enough for me to start speaking up and reclaiming space in yoga land.*

– Vikramjeet Singh, yoga teacher and educator

Microaggressions and weaponising the BIPOC community's lived experience

When people of colour acknowledge the many ways that racism shows up in yoga, we are usually met with responses that downplay our experiences. Here are some (real) examples of such responses that people in my community have experienced:

- **'We are all one, stop bringing race into it,'** which overlooks the struggles faced by people from marginalised racial backgrounds.

- **'Stop playing the victim,'** which dismisses discussions about disrespectful yoga practices.
- **'You're gatekeeping yoga,'** which is an accusation that can be made when individuals from marginalised backgrounds try to teach respectful cultural practices.
- **'Yoga has evolved, it's not positive to keep bringing up the past,'** is a response that ignores the current issues that yoga faces.

It is also common for individuals to tell people from the BIPOC community that they are not very 'yogic' or 'zen' for bringing up issues regarding race and yoga. Personally, I have received multiple comments via social media telling me that I am creating a divide, or that I'm racist by raising awareness around these issues with yoga. I have heard from other BIPOC yoga teachers that they have experienced the same feedback when voicing concerns. This is again problematic because it is essentially a way of avoiding the work that needs to be done to make yoga accessible for all. The divide in yoga clearly exists, and the goal of these discussions (and this book!) is to encourage us all to do the work to bridge that gap, so we can ensure that everyone, regardless of their background, has equal access to the practice.

Yoga and lived experiences from marginalised communities

The following pages are dedicated to the voices of people from marginalised communities, whose experiences are so often left unheard within the modern yoga space.

> *'The difference between myself and others has never been starker than in a yoga class. In one class I went to, I noticed everyone was white, slender and agile. They looked natural, like they are meant to be there. When I looked at myself in the mirror all I saw was that my knees knocked together when I stood, and even though I'm trying not to, my default position is slouched. I'm so much shorter and larger than everyone else. I'm the only South Asian in the room. As the instructor walks around, I realise*

I am sweating, and anxious that she may come up to me. My fears are made true when she stands in front of me and pushes my shoulders down moving my whole body towards the floor. It feels unnatural, uncomfortable, and not right. So I tell her I can't. It takes her a few more moments to stop what she is doing. Then she points at the woman in front of me, who has a wonderful posture, and a slender toned body and says, "You need to do it how she's doing it." I wanted to say, "I can't, that's not how my body moves," but I couldn't bring myself to.'

– Nadiya Hussain, yoga student

'I decided to start practising yoga to achieve inner peace and personal growth. However, as I further researched the practice, I noticed a disturbing trend of cultural appropriation and whitewashing. There was also hyper-sexualization, with no space for the disabled or plus-sized people. Additionally, it seemed incongruent to me that the practice of yoga originated in India and could be so heavily dominated by Anglo-Americans in the United States. As a proud Puerto Rican and "Person of Colour", I felt a sense of discomfort and unease with this erasure of yoga's cultural roots. Therefore, I consciously rejected any participation in the appropriation of yoga and pledged to honour its origins and cultural significance. Learning that yoga is a lifelong daily practise of the mind, body, and spirit that one can do at any moment and that it shouldn't be gatekept is a lesson that should be shouted from the rooftops.'

– Allicette Torres, yoga student

'As a mixed Indigenous person from Abya Yala [one of several names Indigenous people have for the 'Americas' or 'the West'] *seeing the varying degrees of cultural appropriation, racism and microaggressions, and the erasure of Indigenous Indian spirituality and culture (which yoga is birthed from) in yoga spaces led by white women and white men is infuriating and unfortunately, also the 'norm'. This entitlement by white people – or as we know it in BIPOC spaces: 'the audacity of caucasity' – has led to many Black, Brown, and Asian folks feeling unwelcomed and uncomfortable in yoga spaces. It is so normalized for white*

folks to absorb our cultures, wisdom, and spiritualities as if they were their own. This is a product of colonization and the spread of white supremacy. They then sell our cultures to the public with a different face and a different taste that they know will be more digestible to their own white communities. I am a Taino-Borikua woman from the Caribbean Island of Boriken, also known as Puerto Rico. The Caribbean is where European invasion, also known as colonization, began in 1492 with the arrival of Columbus to the ancestral lands of the Taino people, the Greater Antilles. The story goes that he was lost at sea, looking for India but instead found himself stranded in the Caribbean Ocean and was saved by the Taino Arawak people. This was the beginning of a horror story, of genocide, enslavement, of subjugation, and the stripping of culture and language. The violent attempts at breaking a people, a nation who are not broken and still resist today. Although Columbus did not make it to India, other European invaders certainly did and have left their scars. India's most brutal experience of colonization was not by that of an Italian man whose terrorism was funded by Spain, but by the British Empire who ravished the land. However, within the struggle, there has always been resistance. Seeing Indian people take back yoga and decolonize what has been colonized within their culture, is phenomenal and empowering.'

'Bonded by a history of colonization, and the ways that it persists today, the Taino people and Indian people can inspire each other in our contemporary struggles against the theft of our cultures and spiritual wisdom.'

– Ra Ruiz León, yoga student

'I grew up learning yoga through the spirituality of the practice. I would go to the temple every Sunday and I would learn parts of the Bhagavad Gita *while we were there. If we weren't at the temple, we would practice* kirtan *(group chanting of mantras). These experiences introduced me to yoga via wisdom, meditation, and non-attachment. However, the yoga practiced in studios focussed on movement, and it felt disconnected from my upbringing. Discovering that both practices were meant to be the same thing, or came from the same place, was a bit of a journey. After I left*

home, I realised I was trying to find a place where yoga felt similar to the way I practiced growing up, or even a yoga environment that felt similar, but there was always a disconnect. I just did not feel like it was similar at all.'

– Tejal Patel, yoga teacher

'During my teacher training, I sought work experience to prepare myself for after my course was finished. I found an opportunity at a popular yoga centre that was looking for Karma yogis, offering free classes in exchange for working at the reception desk. Initially, this seemed like a great fit.

However, after my first few shifts, I quickly realised this environment was not for me. One of the managers barely acknowledged me. The centre's culture felt exclusive and unwelcoming. The majority of the popular teachers were friends with the manager, and they all seemed to be white, able-bodied women from similar backgrounds. They would dominate the front row in popular classes, performing advanced postures and socialising only within their clique.

There was no effort to make me feel included. Another time, someone pointed to the book I was reading during my shift, The Haṭha Yoga Pradīpikā, *a fundamental and classic yoga text, and dismissively asked, "What is that?"*

The centre emphasised physical postures over the holistic aspects of yoga. Only the physically strong and privileged got the top spots, and teachers had to undergo rigorous physical training just to lead a basic class. I lasted a month before making my excuses and leaving.'

– Anonymous

'Nestled along the pristine shores of Kerala is a tranquil seaside town called Kovalam, where the rhythmic waves whisper tales of serenity and the golden sands cradle moments of bliss.

In August of 2009, it was where I chose to embark on a transformative journey that led me to qualify as a yoga teacher after practising for over 20 years. The essence of yoga lies not just in the physical postures but in the profound philosophy that guides a holistic way of life. However, as I traverse the modern yoga landscape, it becomes glaringly apparent that the industry needs a shift – a shift towards embracing diversity and cultural authenticity.

In the West, yoga has often been packaged and presented in a limited way, depicting a singular body type as the epitome of practice. This not only excludes a multitude of individuals but also perpetuates a narrow perception of what a yogi should look like. The hyper-sexualisation of yoga anatomy further distances the practice from its true purpose, reducing it to a mere physical pursuit. As a yoga teacher, I am passionate about dismantling these stereotypes and fostering an inclusive space that celebrates bodies of all shapes, sizes, and colours.

Moreover, the appropriation of yoga includes a disregard for its linguistic and cultural roots. Many in the West neglect the Sanskrit names of poses, dismissing them as mere jargon. Yet, the sacredness of these names holds the key to understanding the deeper spiritual dimensions of yoga. It is disheartening to witness the dilution of yoga into a mere fitness trend when its essence lies in providing a roadmap for ethical living, both as individuals and as members of a community.

Drawing a parallel to ancient Asian martial arts practices, one can observe a stark difference in the approach to preservation. Martial arts communities adhere to strict protocols, ensuring the sacredness of their teachings. It is not about gatekeeping but preserving the cultural integrity and wisdom embedded in these practices. Yoga, with its rich history and profound teachings, deserves a similar reverence. It's time for the yoga and wellness industry to shift its focus from commercialisation to cultural preservation, embracing the true essence of yoga as a guide to living ethically and harmoniously.'

– Sima Kumar, yoga teacher

Summary

Hopefully you'll now understand some of the reasons why it's valuable to strive for an authentic yoga practice. Yoga should be accessible for everyone, no matter their body type, background or culture. By being aware of the emphasis on physical postures or cultural appropriation in modern yoga, we can appreciate the true essence of the ancient tradition. This way, we can all enjoy the benefits that yoga brings.

Yoga isn't a practice that should be gatekept for the 'elite' and shouldn't be marketed as a luxury, making it exclusionary. Its ancient roots contain the most insightful teachings and tools that we should all have access to. There is so much we can do to ensure that we support diversity when it comes to representation, accessibility and inclusivity so that we are all accepted for who we are. As a community, it is important to recognise how we are going to show up in these spaces to ensure we receive the most fulfilling experience from yoga.

When we empower ourselves through these challenging conversations, we begin to empower others, too. Soon these conversations will no longer be overlooked, and it will be inevitable that we will have them, because people like you and I will act to make yoga a safe and inclusive practice.

Systemic racism in yoga is a complex issue that should be addressed with awareness, empathy and a commitment to anti-racism work. Each of us has a duty to acknowledge these challenges at the same time as creating inclusivity and equality in yoga communities. The onus of representation shouldn't solely rest on people of colour. This work makes us deeply vulnerable and speaking out is not always met with kindness.

The conversations around representation in yoga can be challenging and complicated but they're essential to have, so that yoga is able to serve everyone in our society.

A moment of introspection

Have you encountered racism in yoga or wellness spaces?
If yes, consider the following:

- How have you dealt with these experiences?
- How do you take care of yourself in these situations?
- Do you have people who can support you during these times?
- What does a safe and inclusive environment *look* and *feel* like to you?

→

If no, consider the following:

- Have you noticed any instances where others might have experienced racism or exclusion in these spaces?
- What's one thing you can do to help support people who have experienced racism or exclusion in these spaces?

I then encourage you to reflect on the 'no' questions above, even if you do not identify as BIPOC and/or have never experienced racism in yoga. This is because this exercise may help to shift your perspective from *centring yourself* to *elevating and uplifting BIPOC voices*. Just because exclusion in yoga may not be your lived experience, it doesn't mean you can't use your place of privilege to advocate for change.

Let's take a moment to reflect on our privileges and challenges in yoga. Recognising them helps us understand where we stand and how we can support our communities. Here are mine:

Privileges

- Affording classes
- Having an education
- Being somewhat flexible

Challenges

- Not being completely able-bodied
- Dealing with mental health conditions
- Being a person of colour

What are yours? Feel free to jot them down here or on a separate piece of paper.

Part Two

The foundations of yoga and a very brief history

Now that we're familiar with the issues that surround yoga today, it's time for us to take a look back at yoga's history to see where it all began. Exploring yoga's origins in this way offers us the opportunity to engage with yoga's broader cultural heritage and deep traditions. Understanding this wider history and context is an important step in paving the way for a more authentic and meaningful yoga practice. So, let's begin by taking stock of some (very normal!) questions that might be popping up for you right now.

Q. Is the history of yoga complicated?

A. In short, yes. The history of yoga is very complicated. However, I'm not here to discuss every detail of history; we would never have time for that. For ease of understanding, I will be compressing the history of yoga *a lot*. I have focused purely on the essential information that will help us place everything we've discussed so far into its wider context. I've also focused on highlighting the pivotal fragments of history that make up yoga today, as I want you to have this key information to support you in cultivating a more authentic practice moving forwards. There is, of course, far more to the history of yoga than we'll have space to discuss here, so I encourage you to take your research further in your own time.

Q. Is the history of yoga relevant to my practice now?

A. Yes. Learning about the history of yoga will help you develop a deeper respect for yoga's cultural and spiritual significance, which you can bring to your practice today. Understanding yoga's origins will show you how yoga has so much more to offer than physical poses, and this understanding will help you appreciate and engage with yoga in a more meaningful way.

In addition, learning about – and remaining aware of – the historical marginalisation of certain groups within yoga will help you understand the importance of continuing to advocate for inclusivity and diversity in yoga communities today.

Q. Is the history of yoga controversial?

A. Yes! This is mainly because the practice has been around for so long and it has been interpreted in many ways. The origins are constantly up for debate among scholars and, although it is proven that the practice originated in the Indian subcontinent, identifying its exact beginnings is challenging. It's important to acknowledge therefore that yoga is a shared heritage that is inclusive and encourages collective healing and liberation, so approaching the history of yoga with this open mind would be helpful. This open approach to the history will also help ensure that your journey isn't overly complicated.

I'm not a scholar, but I'm sharing with you the knowledge I've gathered through my extensive research and study. I also want to highlight that although controversies around the history of yoga exist, they do not devalue yoga as a practice that can aid us with our mental, physical and emotional well-being.

In **Part 2**, we'll be looking at the following:

1. **A brief timeline of the history of yoga** – An overview of yoga's development over the years.
2. **The meaning of yoga** – We'll unpack what's at the heart of yogic teaching.
3. **Significant literature in yoga** – We'll discuss yogic texts, yogic scriptures and yogic epics, and I'll provide you with an overview of a few key pieces of yogic literature.
4. **Significant gurus of yoga** – We'll discuss the role of the guru in yoga and I'll give you an introduction to some of the most significant gurus in yoga's history.

1

A brief timeline of the history of yoga

I think it's important to provide a general overview of yoga's development over the years, so I have pieced together a timeline for us to use. It is not essential to memorise all the information in this chapter (don't worry!), but it's helpful background knowledge to skim through, and it is an important part of telling the story of yoga.

Please note that the exact dates are debatable because understanding ancient India's history is a complex task.* Dates have often become lost as Indian knowledge and traditions have historically been transmitted through **guru-shishya paramparā** ('conversations between students and teachers'), inscriptions in mandirs (temples) and manuscripts. Holding on to dates via oral history (i.e. through student and teacher conversations) is tough and information written down was often recorded on palm leaves, which inevitably decomposed – hence why accurate dates are challenging to pinpoint.

However, yoga has survived because of the retelling of the teachings in these forms, and luckily, we can link many of the pieces of the tradition together. So, let's look now at a rough outline of developments in yoga's history. For ease, I have categorised the stages of yoga into four major periods (although you can certainly find more if you wish to look deeper).

These four key periods in yoga's history are: the **Vedic Age**, the **Classical Age**, the **Post-Classical Age** and the **Modern Age**.

* Disclaimer: Pinpointing exact dates is challenging because many of these texts were passed down orally for generations before being written down much later. However, we do know that the **Vedas** are the oldest texts referenced here. Since scholars have proposed a wide range of dates, the periods mentioned in this chapter should be viewed as rough estimates based on my research from various sources. I've left out specific dates for the eras because there are many differing timelines found in books and online.

1. Vedic Age

During this period, the earliest known texts relating to Hinduism emerged, called the **Vedas** (**veda** meaning 'knowledge'). The **Vedas** are comprised of four parts: Rig Veda, Yajurveda, Samaveda and Atharvaveda. These **Vedas** contain songs, hymns, **mantras**, guidance on everyday life, rituals and knowledge of higher wisdom.

The **Vedas** describe Hinduism as a way of life (with yoga at the core of Hinduism). The **Vedas** therefore serve as the foundation for the principles and techniques that are integral to modern yoga practices. The **Vedas** also encourage and promote yoga as a spiritual discipline.

2. Classical Age

During this period, Sage Patañjali compiled *The Yoga Sūtras of Patañjali* (see more on p. 85), in which he systematically organised the practice of yoga into **Aṣṭāṅga** (an eight-limbed path) to lead us to **samādhi** (a state of bliss). The **sūtras** still serve as a way of navigating through life; however, the principles seem to have been lost in modern yoga.

3. Post-Classical Age

Sub-traditions of yoga emerged during this period, including **Haṭha** yoga (body techniques) and **Tantra** yoga (rituals and **mantras**). Two more key texts were written during this period: the *Haṭha Yoga Pradīpikā* and *Gheranda Samhita*. In these texts we see more emphasis on the hidden powers of the body and gurus demonstrated how we can prolong life using advanced yogic practices.

4. Modern Age

Yoga in its present form was introduced to the Western world by scholarly gurus like Swami Vivekananda (see more on p. 95) after India's long period of colonisation.

The intention of introducing yoga to the Western world was to make individuals in the West more spiritually aware. However, this Modern Age has seen the Western world adapt to a 'postural yoga' with a focus on **āsana** – i.e. the modern yoga we commonly see today. Forms of yoga such as **Aṣṭāṅga** (often styled as Ashtanga), **Iyengar** and **Vinyāsa** became popular, and yoga became known as a holistic system for well-being.

2

The roots of yoga

Yoga's roots remain deeply grounded in the ancient wisdom and spiritual traditions of India.

It's difficult to place exact dates on when the practice originated, but scholars generally estimate that initial evidence of yoga can be found around five thousand years ago. We'll be looking at an overview of the meaning behind yoga's roots in this chapter.

Yoga and Hinduism

Yoga is deeply rooted in Hinduism and has strong connections to the religious and philosophical traditions of India. While there are religious roots to yoga, it is *essential* to note that yoga is practised by people of many faiths and backgrounds all over the world, and the practice is not limited to Hindus only. Yoga has historically been linked to other faiths including Buddhism, Jainism and Sikhism.

However, I'm acknowledging the link to yoga's Hindu roots now because yoga's teachings draw upon philosophies that are central to Hinduism, and so it's useful to understand this for a sense of wider context.

Hinduism teaches that there are six schools of philosophy, which are often referred to as **Ṣaḍdarśana**. These schools of philosophy include:

1. **Sāṃkhya**
2. **Yoga**
3. **Nyāya**
4. **Vaiśeṣika**
5. **Pūrva Mīmāmsā**
6. **Vedānta**

We can therefore see here that **Yoga** is one school of thought within Hinduism. It's interesting to understand too that **Yoga** as a concept is actually based on the practical implementation of **Vedānta** and **Sāṃkhya**, which are two other key schools of thought from this list.

So, in summary, everything that we'll be exploring within this book will mainly be within the context of these three schools of philosophy that are integral to Hinduism.

The meaning of yoga

The word 'yoga' is derived from the Sanskrit root **yuj**, which means 'to yoke'. The most common translation of the term 'yoga' in the Western world is 'union' and, in this context, many people believe that yoga means to yoke ('join') your mind to your body.

However, according to yogic tradition, the true purpose of yoga is actually to create union of **shiva** (consciousness) and **shakti** (energy). During this process of union, yoga as a practice guides us towards becoming more in touch with the nature of our true Self (see box below). You see, the outside world is full of constant distractions that can make it virtually impossible for us to get to know ourselves, but yoga gives us the tools we need to help us manage these external factors so that we can turn inwards and focus on the Self.

Getting closer to our Self will allow us to live in balance and harmony, and will ultimately free us from suffering and lead us to **mokṣa*** (liberation), which is at the heart of what yoga is teaching us. When a person achieves **mokṣa**, they have a true understanding of the Self and a profound state of inner stillness. In turn, they have achieved **samādhi** (eternal bliss).

Although exploring yoga as a means of therapy or to heal the body is very valid, these purposes and their benefits are secondary to practising yoga with the aim of attaining **mokṣa**, which is the ultimate goal.

* **Mokṣa:** Before we dive into this term and others like it that will pop up going forwards, it's helpful to know that when you see any terms with this 'ṣ', it's pronounced 'sh' instead of 's'. Remember, as discussed in the section on 'Pronunciation and common Sanskrit terms' on p. 27, understanding these pronunciation nuances helps us differentiate between words that might seem similar otherwise.

The Self

When we are learning the practice of yoga, the Self (also referred to as our **ātman** (soul)) will be referenced regularly. But what do we mean by this?

The Self refers to the true nature or essence of us as an individual. It goes beyond the Physical Body and beyond our thoughts and emotions. As we engage with yogic practices (as outlined in **Part 3**) we begin the journey of transcending and letting go of our ego, physical attachments and our fixation on worldly desires that may limit us, so that we can move closer to – and focus on – our Self. Focusing inwards and coming closer to our Self leads us closer to **mokṣa**.

The cycle of saṃsāra and achieving mokṣa

As **mokṣa** is the ultimate goal of yoga, I think it'd be helpful to dig a little deeper into what we mean by this.

Mokṣa is often referred to in yoga as the 'liberation' from the cycle of birth, life, death and rebirth; this cycle is called **saṃsāra** (think reincarnation). We can only escape **saṃsāra** when we have been able to transcend our ego, our physical attachments and our fixation on other worldly desires and pleasures. In other words, when we have achieved an understanding of the Self.

Avidyā (ignorance) and **rāga** (attachment) keep us trapped in this cycle of **saṃsāra** because they hold us back from understanding the truth that nothing is permanent. Many of us therefore remain attached to the material world and ego, which keeps us far from the Self. This means we are not released from **saṃsāra**, so we keep coming back through rebirth in various forms, rather than achieving liberation and leaving the cycle.

There are two other strong forces that keep us stuck in this loop and would be useful to know about: **karma** and **saṃskāra**. Let's look at both in turn.

1. **Karma** is the law of cause and effect where every thought, intention and action results in consequences. Yogic philosophy suggests that we are all responsible for our own **karma**. Our

karma is connected to the cycle of **saṃsāra** because the consequences of our actions in our current and past lives determine our experiences in future lives. If we have given in to worldly pleasures in a previous life, for example, then it means that we have not yet transcended physical attachments and understood the truth of impermanence that is required to break free from the cycle and achieve **mokṣa**.

2. **Saṃskāra** are imprints or impressions that are stored in our subconscious mind as a result of our past actions, thoughts and experiences. These **saṃskāra** then influence our thoughts, actions and behaviours in the present and future. We can accumulate positive and negative **saṃskāra** that contribute to us having healthy or unhealthy patterns moving forwards. **Saṃskāra** binds us to the cycle of **saṃsāra** because when we act on unhealthy impressions, we reinforce attachment to the material world, which keeps us far from the Self and **mokṣa**.

The practices that yoga provides us with (and which we'll discuss in **Part 3**) guide us through transcending our physical and worldly attachments. This brings us closer to the Self and to freeing ourselves from the suffering of **saṃsāra**, so that we can attain liberation and eternal bliss.

The meaning of yoga: a note on interpretations

I've now given you an overview of the meaning of yoga, and I think most teachers would broadly agree on this. However, as we continue to dig down further into yoga's meaning throughout the rest of the book, it's important for us to acknowledge and understand that there are many, *many* different ways that meaning in yoga can be interpreted further. There is definitely not one simple way of understanding yoga's teachings.

The importance of being open to different interpretations within yoga is by no means a new concept. In fact, this openness is even demonstrated in the teachings from ancient history as the Sanskrit scholar Pāṇini reflected on the several meanings available for the term **yuj** (the Sanskrit root word from which 'yoga' is derived). Pāṇini highlights the following possible interpretations:

- **Yujir Yoge** – Union merger or to join your soul with your higher Self.
- **Yuj Samyamane** – The practice of inner discipline.
- **Yuj Samādhau** – To put together or to integrate by using yogic practices and being free from attachment.

Therefore, the meaning of yoga and the different ways that yoga can be interpreted is vast and broad, and that's something we should remember. But what does this mean in real terms? It means that we should approach the various interpretations of yoga with an open mind and a desire to learn. By being open to exploring classical texts, considering different philosophical viewpoints and engaging in your own practice, you'll gradually uncover how yoga can enrich your own everyday life in a way that feels meaningful to you.

3

Significant literature in yoga

The core literature of yoga contains what are considered to be the 'rules', if you like, of yoga. Not all texts of yoga could be preserved (and some teachings were passed down orally), so acknowledging the ones that remain helps to ensure that we can connect to the true origins while integrating timeless wisdom. Although many of the core texts of yoga were originally written in Sanskrit or other languages of yoga, a lot of them have been translated, interpreted and made accessible in the modern day.

Understanding the foundations of yoga through the literature available will help you see what yoga has to offer beyond the physical poses, and help you embrace yoga for the holistic lifestyle it really is. Therefore, it's helpful to engage with the literature of yoga while building an authentic practice.

The core literature of yoga can be split into three main categories:

1. **Yogic texts** are the foundational texts of yoga. They offer guidelines on how to implement and incorporate yogic techniques, insights and philosophy, often with detailed instructions on how to practise. Essentially, they contain the yogic teachings to help us break free from suffering (i.e. the cycle of **saṃsāra**, see p. 79) and progress on our path to enlightenment.* Examples include *The Yoga Sūtras of Patañjali* (see p. 85) and the *Haṭha Yoga Pradīpikā* (see p. 86).
2. **Yogic scriptures** share common ground with yogic texts in that they contain teachings that are relevant to yoga. However, they also explore a wider range of religious teachings, insights, stories, prayers and rituals that go beyond the teachings of yoga. An example of a yogic scripture is the *Bhagavad Gita* (see p. 87)

* Enlightenment: Often equated with **mokṣa**, enlightenment is the freedom or liberation from the cycle of birth, death and rebirth (**saṃsāra**). It is where we reach an eternal state of bliss otherwise known as **samādhi**.

3. **Epics or 'Itihāsa'** refer to the ancient texts of India. These epics hold information that serve as the foundation of what yoga represents at its very core, as these epics encapsulate the cultural, spiritual and moral values of Hinduism that lead us to live a more conscious life. The epics do refer to yogic philosophy, but they don't directly dive into yogic practices. The two major epics are the *Rāmāyana* (see p. 90) and the *Mahābhārata* (see p. 90).

How can we spot if we're reading a reliable translation of a text?

As most of the core texts of yoga were written in Sanskrit (or other languages of yoga) there are many English translations and interpretations available. Understanding the authenticity and reliability of these translations can be difficult, but it's not impossible. Here are some things to consider:

- **References** – Pay attention to whether the translator refers to the original texts and authentic sources. If they do, this ensures that the translation stays true to the essence of the teachings.
- **Clarity** – If the text is too complex, it might be challenging to grasp the teachings, especially as a beginner. Find translations that use clear and straightforward language.
- **Comparison** – It's always worth comparing various translations of the same text to see if they all align in terms of the original meaning and intent. If they do, it's more than likely a reliable translation.
- **Reviews** – Check to see if there have been reviews or recommendations for translations from experts or authentic figures in the yoga world.

Why do so few practitioners understand key yogic texts?

I believe that there are several reasons why so few yoga practitioners understand and engage with yogic texts.

First, I think for many people the idea of picking up a spiritual book alongside their yoga practice feels unfamiliar or has simply never occurred to them before. This is completely understandable given that many people approach yoga purely as a physical exercise, so diving into spiritual texts alongside this physical exercise might not seem like an obvious step.

Another challenge that one might face is feeling overwhelmed by the sheer amount of reading material available. The lists of recommended reading often handed out at yoga teacher training courses can seem intimidating, so it's easy to feel lost.

In addition, the idea of deciphering yogic texts that date back centuries can feel like a daunting task in itself. The translated texts are often weighty in both content and size, packed with profound teachings that might seem out of reach. Traditionally, yogis would learn from their guru, who would help them navigate yogic texts. But finding an authentic teacher to work with you on this today isn't always feasible, whether that's due to financial constraints or simply not being able to locate an authentic teacher to work with. Without guidance on how to decipher these ancient texts, the task can feel too much.

But there are key yoga texts that I'd recommend for beginners to start with and, luckily for you, this is exactly what we'll be covering in this chapter. I will suggest three beginner texts* of yoga and then I'll introduce you to two of India's greatest epics. (There are then many, many more texts available of course, but I'll leave you to explore these at your own pace.)

Three key pieces of yogic literature for beginners

I've chosen these three particular texts from the wide collection of yogic literature available because I think they work especially well as foundational guides. They provide insight into the very essence of

* To keep things simple, I've used the term 'texts' throughout, but please remember that the *Bhagavad Gita* is a yogic scripture. To help you keep track, I've noted 'text' or 'scripture' next to each piece of literature.

yoga and its application in modern-day practice. By exploring these texts, you'll encounter concepts across yoga practices, philosophy and principles that can form the basis of your yoga journey. I'm going to give you an overview of each one now to act as an entry point. So, let's get into them...

We will be exploring elements of all three texts in **Part 3**, but I do strongly encourage you to dive into the complete versions of these texts at your own pace (these overviews aren't by any means a full interpretation).

Also, please don't be put off if these texts are completely new to you. I am constantly studying them and make no claim to being a master of yoga or having *fully* learned and understood all of them. Yoga is a lifelong journey and a lifelong practice so, no matter how many years of teaching experience or practice you have under your belt, we're all still learning.

1. The Yoga Sūtras of Patañjali (yogic text)

This is one of the most influential texts of yoga and consists of a collection of 196 **sūtras*** (aphorisms). These **sūtras** highlight the most basic and fundamental teachings of yoga, which have been scripted into short verses and organised into four parts: Samādhi Pāda, Sādhanā Pāda, Vibhūti Pāda and Kaivalya Pāda. The purpose of each **sūtra** is for it to be memorised and applied, rather than for a practitioner to read the entire text as a narrative.

The Yoga Sūtras of Patañjali is introduced quite frequently to beginners, particularly in teacher training, but it's actually a fairly complex text so it isn't always easy to understand without guidance. However, we'll be working through some of the teachings from this text in **Part 3**, so we'll unpack them together. This includes the principles and practices of **Rāja** yoga (a key path of yoga, see p. 125), which helps guide practitioners to attaining inner peace, self-awareness and enlightenment through yogic practices.

* **Sūtra:** In Indian literary tradition, a **sūtra** is a concise statement or verse linked to philosophical and spiritual teachings. These are often short and memorable, serving as guiding principles. In the context of yoga, **sūtras** refer to a collection of verses that outline the philosophy and practices of yoga. They provide a clear and compact framework for understanding yoga's principles.

Another key part of this text that we'll be exploring together in **Part 3** is the eight limbs of yoga (see p. 150), as this can be a great place for beginners to start. The eight limbs represent eight practices based on observations and behaviours which, when consistently applied, are designed to support your spiritual journey to enlightenment. The eight principles or limbs are: **yamas** (our behaviours), **niyamas** (self-observances), **āsana** (physical postures), **prāṇāyāma** (breath control), **pratyāhāra** (influence of senses), **dhāraṇā** (concentration of the mind), **dhyāna** (meditation) and **samādhi** (eternal bliss). These provide us with practical guidance to overcoming obstacles like attachment, fear, ignorance and egoism.

The Yoga Sūtras of Patañjali can be interpreted in many different ways and there are various commentaries and translations available that have been made by scholars and teachers. Please see p. 229 for my translation recommendations.

Did you know...?

The story of how the **sūtras** were recorded is heavily debated. It's believed that they were written over 2500 years ago. Some say the **sūtras** were orally transmitted from guru to student until Sage Patañjali wrote them down. Other people state they were not written down by Patañjali himself but by multiple people under the 'Patañjali lineage'. The **sūtras** have been analysed and examined by many people up to the present day but, regardless of their complex history, they play a key part in practising yoga.

2. Haṭha Yoga Pradīpikā (yogic text)

This text offers practical guidelines for **Haṭha** yoga. Originally written in Sanskrit and later translated into English, it is believed to have been composed in the 15th century. The writer, Swami Swatmarama, outlines the foundational principles of **Haṭha** yoga that guide practitioners from body awareness to self-awareness (and ultimately lead us to an eternal state of bliss – **samādhi**).

According to the principles of **Haṭha** yoga, it is essential to purify the body before meditation, so the teachings in the *Haṭha Yoga*

Pradīpikā are centred around preparatory practices that provide us with a foundation for meditation. The text consists of four parts, which cover different aspects of **Haṭha** yoga including: **āsana** (physical postures), **prāṇāyāma** (breath control), **mudrās** (gestures/seals) and **bandhas** (body locks). It also includes guidance on diet and lifestyle and explores spiritual awakening (**kuṇḍalinī**) in detail. I will be referring to this text in **Part 3** as we work through how to practically apply the principles of traditional yoga to your own life.

Did you know...?

Self-discipline is a key theme of authentic yoga, and the *Haṭha Yoga Pradīpikā* is one the oldest and most significant texts that highlights the importance of integrating self-discipline into daily life.

3. Bhagavad Gita (yogic scripture)

The *Bhagavad Gita* ('the *Gita*') forms a key part of the great epic the *Mahābhārata* (see p. 90) but is also itself a key scripture on the supreme science of yoga.* The *Gita* documents the events leading up to a tragic battle set on a battlefield in Kurukshetra (ancient India).

The *Bhagavad Gita* is written in the form of a poem in which there are 700 verses. These verses are a philosophical conversation between Arjuna, a warrior prince, and his charioteer Lord Krishna as the events of the battle begin to unfold. Arjuna experiences a panic attack before the war and is afraid of fighting, which causes him to almost give up. He is reluctant to fight against his relatives and friends who are on the opposing side (the Kauravas). Lord Krishna's teachings in this scripture focus on the battle of the mind that Arjuna experiences.

Essentially, the battle that Arjuna faces mirrors the conflicts that we all experience in our own lives. Lord Krishna represents the divine or a higher power while Arjuna represents us. Krishna passes on his

* Supreme science is a term frequently used to describe yoga. Yoga as a supreme science involves embracing spiritual insights, engaging in transformative practices, and applying philosophical principles. Through this, we cultivate self-awareness, allowing us to uncover the truths that lie within us, leading us to **mokṣa** or liberation.

divine teachings to Arjuna and tells him that he must fulfil his **dharma** (duty), which is a key principle of yoga. Through this conversation, the *Bhagavad Gita* ultimately teaches the importance of 'surrendering' to – or keeping faith in – the divine or a higher power to help cultivate mental and emotional balance.

Although the *Gita* is one of the holiest scriptures in Hinduism, the philosophy it teaches can be applied by anyone, regardless of faith, as the notion of 'surrender' in this sense guides us towards releasing our attachments in every way (to possessions, outcomes and the material world) so we can focus on something bigger than ourselves, as a means of cultivating peace and a deeper sense of purpose in life.

In summary, the *Gita* serves as a guide to yogic living for yoga practitioners all over the world. The wisdom offers timeless guidance on how to better understand ourselves and how to tackle the harsh realities of life, and it is as relevant to children as it is to adults. It provides us with ways of attaining **mokṣa** (liberation) through yogic practices including self-realisation, mind control, selfless action, devotion and meditation. It's for these reasons that we'll be looking at how to apply the knowledge of the *Gita* to our current practice in **Part 3**. (There are many translations and commentaries on the *Gita* and I'll be sharing my favourite recommendation in the Resources section on p. 226.)

Did you know...?

The meaning of *Bhagavad Gita* is 'God's Song' or 'Song of the Lord':

Bhagavad = 'God or a self-realised spiritual teacher'. It can also mean 'devotee'.

Gītam or **gītā** = 'Song or sacred chant'. In Hinduism, **gītā** is usually referred to as a spiritual dialogue and there are many **gītās** that are named after deities or gurus.

The *Bhagavad Gita* is also known as a **Yogaśāstra**, which means 'the scripture that teaches yoga'.

Two of India's greatest epics

The *Mahābhārata* (which includes the *Bhagavad Gita*) and the *Rāmāyana* both help us to understand how the roots of yoga are ingrained in Indian tradition, so I'm choosing to introduce these two to you here. Although these epics aren't specific yoga guides, they serve as the foundation of what yoga represents at its very core. For example, self-realisation and ethical living are central themes in traditional yoga and both the *Mahābhārata* and the *Rāmāyana* play a significant role in providing us with the wisdom, values and insights that we need to align with these themes. They do this by discussing cultural beliefs and by teaching us how to overcome suffering to reach **mokṣa**.

A note to help you understand the two epics

When people think of Hinduism, they think of a religion that has many gods. The truth is that we believe there is one God with many faces in the form of deities. These deities are known as **devās** and **devīs** (gods and goddesses) and they represent different aspects of **Brahman** (supreme reality). Although there are multiple **devās** and **devīs** within this faith, it's believed that **Brahman** transcends all forms and names. Worshipping different **devās** and **devīs** allows everyone to connect to different aspects of this supreme reality that resonates with their personal beliefs (more on this under 'Niyama 5 – Īśvarapraṇidhānā' on p. 161). Saying this, Shiva and Vishnu are two of the most worshipped deities within Hinduism, so let's look at these two now.

Shiva is known as **Adi Yogi** or 'Original Yogi' and is also referred to as **Mahādeva** or 'Great God'. Through his meditative and disciplined nature, Lord Shiva symbolises inner transformation, teaching us the importance of growth and self-discipline, and his devotees worship Shiva for these reasons. He is considered the destroyer of evil, ignorance and attachment, as well as the transformer and creator of new beginnings.

Lord Vishnu is known as the protector of the universe. He is responsible for keeping **dharma** (meaning 'cosmic order' in

→

this context) and for protecting the universe from chaos and destruction. Vishnu is believed to have many avatars and has incarnated on Earth in various forms. His most famous forms are Lord Rama (as seen in the *Rāmāyana*) and Lord Krishna (as seen in the *Gita* on p. 87).

1. Rāmāyana

The *Rāmāyana* is one of two of India's greatest and most treasured epics, where the deeds of Lord Rama (one of the incarnations of Lord Vishnu, see above) are recorded. In short (because the epic is seven books long!), it tells the story of a prince named Rama who is the seventh avatar of Lord Vishnu. After being exiled from Ayodhya (his kingdom), Rama along with Sita (his wife) and Lakshmana (his brother) go to live in the forest. It's not long before the demon king Ravana hears of Sita's beauty and kidnaps her to take her to his kingdom, Lanka. Rama and his brother then go on a challenging journey of triumphs and battles to try and save Sita. Along the way, they receive assistance from an army of monkeys led by Lord Hanuman, who is also a devotee of Rama. With the help of this army, Rama rescues Sita and they all return to Ayodhya, where he becomes ruler again.

The narrative of this epic is focused on **dharma** (duty - and in this sense particularly, moral duty) and themes of good triumphing over evil, honour and duty, and power and loyalty are emphasised throughout the story, which has had a profound impact on yogic philosophy. For yoga practitioners, the *Rāmāyana* can be seen as a spiritual and philosophical guide that teaches valuable life lessons and holds eternal wisdom.

As one of the most significant epics in Hindu literature, the *Rāmāyana* is deeply ingrained in Indian cultural heritage. The themes and messages from the *Rāmāyana* have been kept alive through plays, dance performances, festivals and recitations. Various versions of this story have been told throughout history, but the most influential version has been told by the Indian poet, Valmiki.

2. Mahābhārata

The second of the two greatest epics of India is the *Mahābhārata*, which translates to 'The great tale of the Bharatas'. An Indian sage named Vyasa is believed to have composed this epic in ancient India, and it is one of the largest poems to have ever been written, with over 100,000 verses! (Don't let that put you off though – there are many accessible, shorter and easy-to-read versions out there.)

The narrative is set around a great war, and it depicts the moral dilemmas that are faced by the people who are fighting in it. The story begins with two families, the Pandavas and the Kauravas, who both wish to claim the throne of Hastinapura as their own. After trying to resolve the conflict through diplomatic means and failing, a war breaks out and this is where the great battle of Kurukshetra begins (in comes the *Bhagavad Gita*, as discussed on p. 87).

Many warriors and divine beings participate in this war, which is a conflict between **dharma** (duty or righteousness) and **adharma** (unrighteousness). The war lasts for 18 days and, before it begins, Arjuna seeks guidance from Lord Krishna as he doubts himself. There are many pivotal events during the war and, in the end, the Pandavas transpire as the conquerors. There are many great characters, legends and subplots in the *Mahābhārata*.

For practitioners of yoga, the spiritual wisdom found in the *Mahābhārata* can be drawn upon and integrated into daily life. The characters represent different yogic principles. For example, Arjuna embodies discipline and focus, so by studying these characters we can gain insight into how we can embody these principles of yoga ourselves.

A moment of introspection

Now that you know a bit more about the history of yoga and have become familiar with some of the most significant pieces of literature, let's take a moment to reflect on the following:

- How much of what we've covered in this section resonated with your prior knowledge?
- How might incorporating the wisdom from these ancient sources and having an understanding of yoga's history enhance your personal journey with yoga?
- Which aspect of our exploration intrigued you the most?

4

Significant gurus of yoga

If you've engaged with yoga at all then you've probably heard of the term 'guru'. Gurus still exist and play a key role in yoga today, so it's an important topic to address here. Understanding the significance of gurus will help you as you build to a more authentic practice.

We'll begin with a few basic questions that I always receive about gurus, then I'll introduce you to five of the most influential gurus in history. Let's start.

What is a guru?

A loose translation of the term **guru** is 'dispeller of darkness'. This signifies someone who specialises in spiritual knowledge and who passes this wisdom down to their students, guiding them towards a path of self-awareness and self-realisation.

In yoga and Indian traditions, particularly Hinduism, a guru is a teacher, mentor or guide who has dedicated their life to studying, practising and transmitting yoga in different ways. Traditionally, the contents of yogic texts, including sacred spiritual practices and teachings, would be transmitted orally from guru to student.

In fact, Swami Swatmarama, author of the *Haṭha Yoga Pradīpikā* (see p. 86), even stated that one can only get so far with instructions from books alone. He claimed that to progress in yoga it's essential for you to work with the careful guidance of an experienced teacher. Gurus have been highly regarded throughout Indian history.

Q. Do gurus still exist in yoga today?

A. Yes. Although the term 'guru' is now commonly used in Western spaces as a label for an expert in any field, the yogic gurus I refer to here still play an important role in Indian traditions and Hindu practices.

Gurus continue to impart their wisdom in the modern day and without this knowledge the practice of yoga would lack authenticity. Gurus can be found worldwide, but they hold particular significance in India, where they have a rich history of sharing their wisdom to guide people on their spiritual path.

Q. Is my regular yoga instructor my guru? Can they be?
A. To be called a guru one must have been initiated into something called a **saṃpradāya**, which in simple terms is a tradition through which ancient teachings are passed down from one generation of gurus to their students or followers. Initiation into a **saṃpradāya** often takes the form of a formal ceremony, which can include vows.

While gurus may seem similar to teachers, especially in a Western context, if you have a teacher who hasn't been initiated within a **saṃpradāya**, then this person cannot technically be called a guru, so you could call them your 'spiritual guide' instead. (Both spiritual guides and gurus impart knowledge, but a guru has a deeper spiritual connection to their lineage.)

Of course, the disclaimer here is that if your regular yoga teacher focuses mainly on the physical aspects of yoga (without diving into the deeper spiritual connections the practice has to offer), then they would be seen more as your teacher of **yoga āsana** (yoga poses), rather than your spiritual guide.

Q. Can I practise yoga authentically if I don't have a guru or spiritual guide?
A. In an ideal world, every student of yoga would have a guru or spiritual guide leading them through the practice. However, if you don't have one (as I'm sure is the case for the vast majority of people reading this), don't worry at all. What truly matters is your sincerity and commitment to understanding yoga beyond the physical practice. (In fact, even by simply understanding about gurus and their role in yoga, you are taking another step towards practising yoga more authentically.)

You can also still access the wisdoms and teachings of gurus by yourself. This is because their invaluable insights have been preserved through various means, including written texts (which we'll be touching on now...).

Five significant gurus of yoga

Throughout the history of yoga there have been many great gurus. So many, in fact, that a single book wouldn't be enough to mention them all! So, for now, I'll introduce you to five of the gurus, all native to India, who I believe have had the most significant impact on yoga as it stands today.

You'll soon see, all gurus are connected through the main message of their work: an emphasis on self-awareness and self-realisation through yogic practices. But each guru brings a unique perspective that allows you to deepen your understanding of yoga in a different way. So, as you read through below, see if any of the gurus' insights resonate with you. If they do, then I encourage you to explore the guru's work further.

It's now time to meet the gurus.

1. Patañjali (2nd–4th century BCE)

Let's start by introducing Patañjali, who is one of the most important figures in the history of yoga. There is minimal information available about the guru himself, but we do know that he provided us with some of the most influential texts in yoga's history on the philosophical and practical aspects of yoga.

You may remember the name from earlier as we previously discussed Patañjali's most famous piece of work, *The Yoga Sūtras of Patañjali* (p. 85). This text has shaped our understanding of yoga as a path to spiritual awakening and mastery of the mind, and it also introduced us to the very popular concept of **Aṣṭāṅga**, which is the eight limbs of yoga (explored further in **Part 3**). His work helped contribute to the systematising of yoga into an accessible framework, and his teachings have had a great impact on our understanding of yoga as a practice for self-awareness and self-realisation.

No one knows exactly when Patañjali lived, although it is believed to be around the 2nd-4th century BCE. Despite this, Patañjali's work still remains very relevant to us today and is used and studied by yoga practitioners all over the world. For this reason, it's definitely worth exploring this great guru further.

Numerous researchers have suggested that Patañjali may also have been well-versed in other subjects, such as grammar and **Āyurveda** (more on this on p. 144).

2. Swami Vivekananda (1863–1902)

Next up we have Swami Vivekananda, a Hindu monk who was one of the most famous and influential spiritual leaders of yoga. Born in Calcutta, and spiritual from a very young age, he intricately studied Hindu scriptures, such as epics including the *Rāmāyana* and the *Mahābhārata* (p. 90), while at the same time being exposed to Western philosophy and science. Vivekananda played a crucial role in introducing Hinduism to the Western world.

Vivekananda was determined to show the world that the Indian people would not remain defined or oppressed by European occupiers, despite the colonisation under the British Raj. To highlight this, he began delivering speeches in the USA, and then later in some European countries, too, to spread Hindu teachings on God, **ātman** (soul) and the mind-body connection.

In September 1893, Vivekananda participated in the Parliament of World Religions* and he made it his mission to bring India's traditional heritage and spiritual wealth to a global platform. In his famous speech, he addressed the core principles of **Vedānta**† and introduced yogic teachings and philosophy. He presented Indian culture in its most sophisticated and deepest form, and he hoped to make the world more spiritually aware to help ease suffering and uplift people.

Vivekananda taught that we should apply yogic principles to our daily lives while engaging in our daily responsibilities. He also emphasised the importance of exploring the four paths of yoga mentioned in the *Bhagavad Gita* (p. 87). His spiritual wisdom and teachings made him famous worldwide, and his work has influenced many yoga practitioners, gurus and scholars. Vivekananda's teachings

* The Parliament of World Religions was an organisation that aimed to spread awareness and understanding of different traditions and religions by bringing together religious and spiritual communities. It was a space to discuss topics such as social justice, culture and how to engage with and respect each other's faiths.

† **Vedānta**, meaning 'end of the **Vedas**', is a system of Hindu thought that is based on the teachings of the **Vedas** (the oldest and most sacred texts that form the foundation of Hinduism).

live on today with the Ramakrishna Mission (a religious and spiritual organisation) playing a key role in preserving his teachings. If you decide to explore yoga further, you will no doubt come across many of his books as they remain relevant to our lives today.

Beyond his spiritual contributions, Vivekananda was also known for advocating for the rights of women and minorities. His substantial work and legacy in the world paved the way for other spiritual teachers who sought success in the West, one of whom is the next guru we're going to meet...

3. Śri Tirumalai Krishnamacharya (1888–1989)

Śri Tirumalai Krishnamacharya played a key role in spreading the teachings of yoga and **Āyurveda** (see p. 144) to the Western world, and he was integral to the development of **Aṣṭāṅga** yoga, after it was originally introduced by Patañjali. Krishnamacharya also had a deep interest in using yoga as a healing system to help others with illnesses.

Krishnamacharya's curiosity for learning yogic practices began due to his family's close links to yoga: his first teacher was his father, and the famous yogi Nathamuni* was one of his ancestors. After studying with gurus for years, he was told by his own guru that he should begin spreading the message of yoga himself, so he decided to become a guru.

Krishnamacharya's style of teaching was unique at the time since he tailored the holistic system of yoga to each individual, using techniques from different disciplines of yoga to do this (almost providing bespoke yoga, if you will). He also taught the importance of combining breath with movement and it was from here that **Aṣṭāṅga** yoga, as you may know it today, developed.

Everything Krishnamacharya taught emphasised the therapeutic aspects of yoga as he encouraged people to use yoga as a way of

* **Nathamuni** was a yogi and scholar who contributed to preserving and systematising the ancient teachings of yoga. His work has been significant in transmitting yogic practices such as **āsana** (physical postures), **prāṇāyāma** (breath control) and meditation, which can be found in the text *Yoga Rahasya*.

healing the mind and body. His teachings were mostly based on *The Yoga Sūtras of Patañjali* (p. 85) and the *Yoga Yājñavalkya*.*

Krishnamacharya's teachings were pivotal in shaping the careers of numerous gurus, such as B. K. S. Iyengar† and Pattabhi Jois,‡ who then went on to become influential yoga teachers in the Western world. Krishnamacharya's son, T. K. V. Desikachar, continued his legacy and Desikachar's book *The Heart of Yoga* is used widely among yoga enthusiasts today. I'll be referencing this text a lot as we move through **Part 3**.

4. Swami Sivananda Saraswati (1887–1963)

We don't often hear much about this guru in yoga spaces nowadays, but he was very influential in promoting yoga as a practice for self-development.

Swami Sivananda wasn't always a teacher; during his early years, he pursued a career as a doctor. However, he had always felt a calling to spread the knowledge of spiritual philosophy, so he soon gave up his medical career to follow a spiritual path instead. When Swami Sivananda settled in Rishikesh, India, he began seeking guidance from great gurus of yoga and he practised intensely. Soon after being initiated by his guru (i.e. after being formally accepted as a student), Swami Sivananda started promoting yoga as a practice for self-development. He encouraged individuals to incorporate yogic principles into their daily lives and to embody self-discipline and selfless service.

In 1936, Swami Sivananda established the Divine Life Society to spread his message of yoga as a practice for self-development and to share spiritual literature for free with yoga communities. The organisation continues to spread his legacy today through its ashrams worldwide. Swami Sivananda has written over 200 books that cover topics such as yoga, **Vedānta** philosophy and spirituality. The wisdom and knowledge that Swami Sivananda shared has had a huge impact on many people globally.

* ***Yoga Yājñavalkya*** is an ancient yogic text that discusses integrating various practices of yoga into daily life.

† **B. K. S. Iyengar** was a guru and founder of the system of yoga known as **Iyengar** yoga. This style of yoga focuses on correct alignment with props such as blocks, straps and blankets.

‡ **Pattabhi Jois** was a guru also popular for his work in developing **Aṣṭāṅga** yoga.

5. Paramahansa Yogananda (1893–1952)

This brings us to Paramahansa Yogananda. Born in 1893, Yogananda was a Hindu monk, yoga teacher and author of *Autobiography of a Yogi*, which became a classic spiritual text. In his book, Yogananda describes his own mystical experiences with yoga and his encounters with great sages and saints of yoga.

Yogananda was responsible for introducing yoga in the form of **Kriyā** yoga to the Western world in 1920. He describes **Kriyā** yoga as 'an instrument through which human evolution can be quickened'. In real terms, **Kriyā** yoga is a type of yoga that combines **āsana**, **prāṇāyāma** and meditation techniques.

It was Yogananda's own guru, Swami Śri Yukteswar Giri, who encouraged him to share Eastern spirituality with the West. Yogananda recalls in his book how his guru told him: 'I want you to enter college in Calcutta ... Someday you will go to the West. Its people will be more receptive to India's ancient wisdom if the strange Hindu teacher has a university degree.'

In 1920, Yogananda founded the Self-Realization Fellowship (SRF) to spread the teachings of **Kriyā** yoga and promote spiritual growth. Across the USA and Europe, Yogananda held classes, workshops and lectures in which he encouraged people to cultivate a deep connection with the divine and to explore their spiritual potential.

Although Yogananda died in 1952, his influence remains a large part of traditional yoga. The Self-Realization Fellowship still plays a key part in delivering his teachings today through study groups, classes and temples in their worldwide branches.

Women in yoga

I often hear people discuss the lack of women present in the history of yoga. You may have been wondering this yourself during our discussion of the gurus. If so, let's add some further context to this conversation now because women were, and have always been, an integral part of yoga's history.

Women were actively involved in the practice of yoga (and in other spiritual practices) in ancient times, and yoga was not

→

specific to any gender. Female yogis (also known as **rishikas**) are mentioned in texts as early as the Rig Veda, which is one of the four parts of the **Vedas** (discussed on p. 75). These (female) yogis were valued for their wisdom, knowledge and spiritual attainments.

There have been several women in yoga who have made significant contributions to the development and transmission of yogic teachings. A well-known example is Mirabai, a 16th-century Hindu poet and devotee of Lord Krishna. Mirabai made a great impact on the **Bhakti** (devotional) yoga movement and her influence lives on through her poems and songs to this day.

Women have played and continue to play a huge role in the development and evolution of yoga. However, sadly, as is the case throughout much of history, their contributions have not always been made visible. I therefore highly encourage you to dive deeper into the topic of women in yoga, as there are many fascinating aspects to explore.

Controversies to acknowledge

TRIGGER WARNING: You may find some of this information distressing.

While we are on the topic of the gurus in yoga, I would like to acknowledge the sensitive issue of the gurus who have been accused of sexual abuse and harassment. As much as I don't want this be a part of this text, it is important to mention it for your safety and awareness. I won't be naming the false gurus who have misused their positions, as they do not deserve space in this book, and I do not want their behaviour to take away from our purpose of learning yoga authentically.

It's unfortunate that there have been countless accusations of abuse and harm against some of the leading gurus in yoga, so much so that to some degree the term 'guru' has lost its meaning because of the associations it has. While many accused gurus deny any wrongdoing, the allegations cannot be ignored. Some key yogic texts have authors who have faced accusations, and, with those, I would suggest you use your own judgement on whether you would like their work to be a part of your practice.

It may be a question of asking 'Can the teacher be separated from their teachings?' It's not for me to give you an answer, it's for you to come to your own conclusion about what feels right for you. If certain authors trigger discomfort, there's no pressure to use their books. If you're unsure, then you might like to consider questions such as: 'Are they harmful practices?' 'Do they promote violence and abuse?' and 'Are the teachings in alignment with authentic yoga?' You may be able to gauge this after finishing this book.

Personally, I learned a great deal from some texts only to later discover allegations against the authors. While I was initially hurt and disappointed, I found that many teachings were still authentic and valuable. However, I know other people who struggle to disconnect the author and the work, so they feel more comfortable skipping certain books completely. The choice is yours to make.

Please keep in mind your safety and comfort. My experiences and opinions are shared here to contribute to these ongoing discussions, and I respect your own choice. Discernment is important and doing the work to find out what ways of teaching are genuine while avoiding false gurus is vital for this reason. With that being said, if you're ever exploring the idea of working with a spiritual teacher yourself, then I suggest you be mindful of the following:

1. Avoid committing to their teachings unquestioningly. Instead, do question their teachings and regularly evaluate how they are contributing to your practice.
2. Look out for power plays, such as them not receiving feedback or criticism well, or them manipulating practitioners.
3. No teacher should be hero worshipped in an unhealthy way.

A moment of introspection

Now that we have covered a lot on gurus, I think it's a good idea for us to reflect on the following questions to help you integrate what you've learned into your current practice:

- What new insights have you gained from our discussion of gurus?
- Do you have a guru or spiritual leader in your life currently? If not, does having one appeal to you?
- What aspect of our discussion has intrigued you the most? If you were to research this further then what would be the next step to take?

Part Three

Integrating authenticity into your practice

Now that you're more familiar with the history and origins of yoga, it's time to explore the many *practical* ways that we can practise traditional yoga ourselves.

The goal in **Part 3**, therefore, is to introduce you to elements of traditional yoga that are often overlooked in the modern day. To do this, I'll be breaking down different types of authentic yoga and giving you a variety of practical suggestions for how you can integrate this traditional yoga into your life. You may already have a yoga practice and, if that's the case, then you don't have to give this up. Instead, I encourage you to view this section as a way of learning about new yoga practices, all of which can be adapted and added seamlessly into your current routine to enhance it.

Some of the practices may be completely new to you, and some may sound familiar but might not necessarily be about what you think... As yoga is so broad (I like to think of it as a philosophical umbrella), it can of course be *very* complicated. For example, for each 'type' of yoga that exists, there are thousands of different ways that the teachings and practices can be interpreted and applied by different practitioners. So, how then have I decided what to include here?

Well, in **Part 3** I've chosen to emphasise the aspects of yoga that I believe are the most relevant to beginners, especially from a non-physical perspective. Most yoga books available today tend to emphasise **āsana** (physical poses), as discussed in **Part 1**, so my intention here is to give you practices that are not readily available in your average yoga manual. Be prepared for a mix of accessible and practical exercises – some physical and many not – with some intriguing theory added in along the way, too!

How to approach Part 3

As a newbie to yoga, it's important that you don't overwhelm yourself at this stage while trying out new practices. You might, therefore, find it easiest to briefly flick through the whole of **Part 3** first to see if any sections resonate with you more than others, and if they do then you can start there. If that means beginning with the parts that focus on **āsana**, then so be it. Alternatively, you could immediately pick one specific section at random to read in full and implement the practices from there. Either approach is fine and both will mean you're taking baby steps towards a more authentic practice, which is our goal. Everything provided in **Part 3** offers a way of practising traditional yoga, so there is no right or wrong in terms of where you start and how you approach this.

That being said, you will find that not *all* practices in **Part 3** will necessarily apply to you and your current life right now. I suggest you start with a few exercises first, get used to these, and then only explore more when you're comfortable with the first set. Keep going with practices that work for you and put aside those that don't. This is all part of the process, and it's important to remember to be kind to yourself.

Also, remember that during former ages finding time for **sādhanā*** was easier as people often had more time and could dedicate most of their days to it. Take my grandparents for example, they would devote a large portion of their mornings to **sādhanā**. Nowadays it's almost impossible to find just a few hours per day due to the demands of modern-day living. However, committing to 30 minutes every day or every other day is enough to make a difference in your spiritual growth.

Please note: Whenever you see the lotus symbol ( ) in **Part 3**, this indicates that there will be a practice for you to try. You can revisit any of the practices at your own pace; they don't have to be carried out as you are reading along.

Right, I'm sure this is the part that you've all been waiting for: let's now learn how yoga in its most traditional form can enter your life.

* **Sādhanā** is a daily spiritual practice that involves working on yourself through yogic practices. The meaning of the term **sādhanā** is 'spiritual discipline' and in this sense, we carry out **sādhanā** to cultivate self-awareness, transcend the ego and equip ourselves with knowledge.

A note on terminology

A reminder that when I say 'traditional yoga' I'm talking about using the practice of yoga as a tool for self-awareness and mindfulness in order to reach **mokṣa** (liberation), as discussed on p. 79. The terms 'classical yoga', 'authentic yoga' and 'respectful yoga' also mean the same thing in this context. All the practices discussed in **Part 3** fall under the category of traditional yoga.

I will also be discussing different 'styles' or 'types' of yoga, by which I mean the different forms of yoga that have developed over time. Many forms of yoga have evolved as yoga's teachings have been interpreted in different ways by different people over the years (for instance, see p. 74 for more on the history of yoga). **Haṭha**, **Iyengar** and **Aṣṭāṅga** are all examples of different styles or types of yoga, for example.

In **Part 3**, we'll be exploring the following:

1. **Three key yogic teachings** – Three principles from the philosophy of yoga to help you remember the purpose of yoga as you explore new things.
2. **Types or styles of yoga** – An overview of the classical styles of yoga, with practices and tips.
3. **Traditional yoga: the four key mārgas** – **Mārga** means 'path' in Sanskrit, so we'll be looking at the four main paths of yoga according to the key yogic text the *Bhagavad Gita*.
4. **Traditional yoga: Haṭha yoga** – Exploring what **Haṭha** yoga encompasses, including some tips on what to expect from a traditional **Haṭha** yoga practice.
5. **A note on chakras** – An overview of the significance of **chakras** in yoga (since the true meaning is often misunderstood in the Western world).
6. **Traditional yoga: Aṣṭāṅga yoga** – An introduction to the eightfold path of yoga, otherwise known as **Aṣṭāṅga** yoga. Each of the eight limbs will be covered in turn in the following chapters.

7. **Limb 1: yamas (our behaviours)** - An outline of the ethical principles in yoga philosophy that guide us to cultivate integrity in our thoughts, actions and relationships.
8. **Limb 2: niyamas (self-observances)** - Exploring the five personal observances that help us to adopt a harmonious lifestyle.
9. **Limb 3: āsana (physical postures)** - Uncovering the true meaning of **āsana**, i.e. understanding the purpose of the physical poses, the benefits and the practical application.
10. **Limb 4: prāṇāyāma (regulation of breath)** - A journey into the breath and how we can use it to foster a balanced state of mind.
11. **Limb 5: pratyāhāra (the influence of our senses)** - Exploring how to control our senses to prepare our body for meditation.
12. **Limb 6: dhāraṇā (concentration of the mind)** - A discussion on the importance of concentrating the mind on one object to prevent it from wandering during meditation.
13. **Limb 7: dhyāna (meditation)** - A brief outline of what the state of **dhyāna** is and how it differs from practices.
14. **Limb 8: samādhi (pure awareness)** - A brief overview of the state of **samādhi**.
15. **Yoga Nidrā: a practice for deep relaxation** - An explanation of **Yoga Nidrā**, including a guided practice.
16. **Studying yogic texts/scriptures** - Details of how to approach studying yogic texts.

1

Three key yogic teachings

To set you up for success, there are three key teachings from yogic philosophy that I would suggest you try to keep in mind when experimenting with the practices in **Part 3**. Think of these as friendly guides. They'll remind you that while yoga practices can be adjusted to fit our modern lifestyles, the core purpose of the practices remains unwavering: to nurture discipline and focus on our journey of spiritual growth as we strive for **mokṣa** (liberation). Remembering these will make it simpler for you to understand the fundamental purpose of any of the different practices you try. Let's look at each in turn.

1. Abhyāsa – Consistent and focused practice leads to a calm mind

Abhyāsa is a major component of yogic philosophy as it encourages us to prioritise a consistent and focused practice as a way to achieve a tranquil mind, which in turn will help us to become a better version of ourselves.

Abhyāsa is mentioned in both the *Bhagavad Gita* (see p. 87) and *The Yoga Sūtras of Patañjali* (see p. 85). In the *Bhagavad Gita*, Lord Krishna reassures Arjuna that the restless mind can be controlled by a dedicated practice, as he advises:

श्रीभगवानुवाच |
असंशयं महाबाहो मनो दुर्निग्रहं चलम् |
अभ्यासेन तु कौन्तेय वैराग्येण च गृह्यते || 35||

śhrī bhagavān uvācha
asanśhayaṁ mahā-bāho mano durnigrahaṁ chalam
abhyāsena tu kaunteya vairāgyeṇa cha gṛihyate

'It is true that the mind is restless and difficult to control. But it can be conquered, Arjuna, through regular practice and detachment.'
– *Bhagavad Gita* (6:35) by Eknath Easwaran*

Abhyāsa means that it is a focus on consistent practice (not a focus on our aspiration of tranquility itself) that ultimately paves the way to our desired outcome. The greater our consistency and dedication to our practice then the easier it will be to overcome any difficulties and to calm the mind. There's no need to worry about the speed of your progress. Instead, simply keep practising and, with time, there's no doubt that you will experience transformation. There is no judgement if you miss days of practice or fall out of routine, though. As long as you come back, show up and keep going, that's all that matters.

So, what does this look like in real terms? The application of **abhyāsa** simply means doing something repeatedly and consistently with the intention of gaining steadiness and control of the mind. It teaches us to persevere, to stay dedicated, to stay committed and to keep trying, even if and when we experience discomfort.

As you move through **Part 3**, and begin experimenting with new practices, I encourage you to stick with the theme of **abhyāsa** as much as you can. This will allow you to approach each new practice you decide to try with a sense of mindfulness and consistency (even through the times when you may find it a struggle!). Approaching each practice in this way means that, over time, these new practices will naturally become a part of your life.

The concept of **abhyāsa** is helpful when it comes to managing our expectations of the term 'practice' in the yoga world, too. This is because it reminds us that 'yoga' does not always equate to **āsana**. Instead, **abhyāsa** promotes mental discipline over physical potential, so adopting **abhyāsa** in your life is a wonderful way for anyone who struggles with **āsana** to practise yoga.

You can practise **abhyāsa** in your yoga through the following:

- **Setting goals** – Start small and create goals that are achievable.

* Along your journey you may come across chapters and verses in this format. These are ways to help readers locate specific teachings or passages in yogic texts and scriptures. In this case, the number 6 here refers to the chapter of the scripture or text, and the 35 refers to the verse.

- **Creating space** – Keep a dedicated space for your practice.
- **Being mindful** – Try to stay present and in the moment in any of your yoga practices.
- **Be open to change** – Every day isn't the same – things change and life happens! Adapt your practice when you need to but stay consistent.
- **Practise with someone** – Seek out a regular class or a teacher so that you can track your progress and be held accountable.

2. Antarāyas – Embrace the obstacles we may encounter in yoga

It's very normal to face challenges and disruptions in our yoga routine. Yoga philosophy teaches us that there are nine obstacles that can arise within us at any time, and these can affect our focus on our yoga journey and hinder our ability to achieve inner peace.

I think it's important to acknowledge these nine obstacles early on in **Part 3** so that we know to expect them. If we understand that these obstacles are an integral part of our yoga practice then we can be prepared to face them with kindness, openness and compassion for ourselves, and with a determination to keep moving forwards, rather than leaning into self-criticism.

In *The Yoga Sūtras of Patañjali* (see p. 85), the nine **antarāyas** in yoga are identified as:

1. **Vyādhi** (mental illness) – When you feel unwell mentally or physically, it can be almost impossible to carry out any task effectively.
2. **Styāna** (mental laziness or procrastination) – Sometimes you might feel like putting off practising because of a lack of enthusiasm or motivation. This can also come across as feeling lethargic.
3. **Saṃśaya** (doubt) – This can manifest as being uncertain or feeling indecisive to the point where you start questioning yourself and your abilities.
4. **Pramāda** (neglect or carelessness) – When you aren't paying attention to your practice because you're too focused on outcomes and eventually park it to one side altogether.

5. **Ālasya** (physical laziness) – Your ability to practise the physical aspects of yoga is affected because you don't feel like you have the energy or motivation.
6. **Avirati** (being distracted by external factors) – You feel distracted by materialistic things. Being attached to sensual pleasures can lead us astray from the yogic path.
7. **Bhrāntidarśana** (false perception) – You are distracted from your yoga journey because you become caught up in thinking (incorrectly!) that you know everything. This is usually due to a lack of intelligence.
8. **Alabdhabhūmikatva** (inability to make progress) – If you haven't seen results (or if you haven't seen what you deem to be big enough results) then you feel like giving up on your yoga because your efforts don't feel like they are being rewarded.
9. **Anavasthitatva** (instability) – Even once you have made progress, it can be difficult to stay consistent with yoga and grow further because you may feel like you have achieved everything already in your practice.

Each obstacle serves as a reminder that it's normal to experience setbacks on your self-improvement journey, so there is no need to be hard on yourself as and when you face them. Some days will be easier than others when it comes to practice, but in the words of Swami Vivekananda: 'Persevere. All progress proceeds by rise and fall.'

The list of obstacles is also an important reminder that yoga isn't always about 'love and light'; yoga is a journey of constant evolution. Embracing the reality that there's always more to learn and overcome is a humbling aspect of the spiritual path of yoga.

Luckily, yoga provides us with many ways that we can overcome these obstacles and I will be sharing many of these with you as we go.* You see, the more you dig into yoga, the more you will discover that it provides us with the answer to almost anything in life. This is what makes gaining a deeper understanding of yoga so enriching. (Feel free to revisit this list at any point as you move through **Part 3**, as I understand it can be a useful reminder that you're not alone.)

* The *Yoga Sūtras of Patañjali* also gives specific details of how to overcome these obstacles (1:34–1:40) if you'd like to explore this further.

3. Puruṣa (true Self) and prakṛti (the nature of existence)

In the chapter in **Part 2** called 'The roots of yoga' (p. 77), we briefly mentioned how yoga serves as the practical implementation of the Hindu school of philosophy, **Sāṃkhya**. **Sāṃkhya** is the belief that the path to liberation comes from self-realisation. Throughout **Part 3**, I'll be introducing you to key concepts from the teachings of **Sāṃkhya** philosophy, so that you can begin to implement them into your current practice for a more authentic yoga experience. But, first, I think it'll be helpful to give you a brief overview of the main ideas of **Sāṃkhya** so you can keep these in mind.

You may be familiar with the Western concepts of 'mind' and 'matter' (for example, there's the common phrase 'mind over matter'). If so, then **Sāṃkhya** is similar in the sense that it embodies a dualistic perspective that consists of two fundamental realities in the universe. (To clarify: when we refer to the 'universe' in this context, we're not referring to an external entity but rather to our inner selves. Within yogic philosophy, the universe is thought of as a core aspect within each of us, which makes our exploration more introspective.) The two realities within **Sāṃkhya** philosophy are:

1. **Puruṣa** (true Self) – This is the part of us that is associated with reality and perception. This is never-changing, and it is the essence of who you are without the influence of external factors. **Puruṣa** always stays the same regardless of what happens in your life. This is your true Self.
2. **Prakṛti** (the nature of existence) – This encompasses the material world, including aspects of ourselves: our mind, body, thoughts and feelings, which are constantly changing and evolving. There are always shifts happening within each of us and the world around us. **Prakṛti** is also described as **māyā** (meaning 'illusion'), which is often seen as the cause of **duḥkha** (suffering). This is because **māyā** suggests that what we perceive as real may not actually be real. Because of **māyā**, things are always changing and that can bring us sadness or suffering.

Yoga teacher and spiritual guide T. K. V. Desikachar summarises the concept of **puruṣa** and **prakṛti** for us as follows: 'Puruṣa is that part of us capable of real seeing and perception. It is not subject to change. Conversely, Prakṛti is subject to constant change and embraces all matter, even our mind, thoughts, feelings, and memories.'

However, the goal of **Sāṃkhya** philosophy is to recognise the difference between these two realities, so that we can move beyond **prakṛti** and become aware of **puruṣa**. It is only when we realise that our **puruṣa** is separate from the **prakṛti** that we can achieve yoga's ultimate goal of **mokṣa** (liberation). When we reach this state of liberation, we are finally free from the cycle of **saṃsāra** (the cycle of birth, death and rebirth) and from **duḥkha**, as we discussed on p. 79.

Practising yoga with the wisdom of **Sāṃkhya** philosophy offers several benefits, especially for beginners. For example, it guides us towards detachment from the material world by teaching us to discern between our Self (**puruṣa**) and the ever-changing material world (**prakṛti**). This helps our perception of reality become clearer, which in turn helps us to navigate life's ups and downs with grace and understanding. As we gradually uncover the unchanging essence of **puruṣa**, beyond the material world, we also experience a sense of inner peace and harmony that comes with being more attuned to our true nature. Both realities, **puruṣa** and **prakṛti**, help us to explore the true nature of our inner selves and our surroundings.

Throughout **Part 3** I will be introducing you to the practices and key concepts of **Sāṃkhya**. As you'll see, these practices are simple yet insightful and help us to look within, and observe our thoughts and emotions with kindness and curiosity.

Having these three key yogic teachings of consistency, obstacles and the Self in mind while you practise yoga is a great first step in adding authenticity to your current practice. A knowledge of these will also aid you greatly in staying grounded and focused on yoga's core principles as you try out different practices in **Part 3**.

2

Types or styles of yoga

Many people enter the world of yoga feeling confused as to which class might suit them best. Speaking from experience, I believe a huge part of this confusion is because there are so many different types of yoga available on the market in the Western world today. Anyone new to the practice is bound to feel lost – I know I did!

As we discussed in **Part 1** (p. 48), yoga's growing popularity in the Western world has led to the creation of new styles of yoga, often driven by business interests. With more types of yoga available there's a greater opportunity for studios to offer more classes (to cater to all the different types of yoga), which makes yoga more profitable. While it's great to see so many styles, it's important to recognise that this commercialisation can sometimes overshadow yoga's traditional teachings and spiritual essence.

We will only be focusing on a selection of the traditional types of yoga in **Part 3**. And, since this is a book for beginners, we'll only be focusing on the traditional types of yoga that are suitable for those new to the practice.

Popular yoga styles

You might have heard of these popular types of classes. As our focus is on traditional styles, we won't be discussing these in detail here, but you may find value in them. Though developed relatively recently, some of these practices, like **Vinyāsa** and **Iyengar**, are deeply rooted in the authentic practice.

- **Vinyāsa** yoga (modern yoga) – A fluid and dynamic style of yoga that links breath with movement. The term **Vinyāsa** often equates to 'flow' in the modern day and teachers have used it to describe the transition from one pose to the next. By weaving this fluidity into the sequence of **āsana**, it's thought →

to cultivate a sense of meditation in motion, where you can find peace and focus while moving through your practice. Although most **Vinyāsa** classes today are fast-paced, 'dynamic' doesn't have to mean rushing through each posture.
- **Yin** yoga (modern yoga) – A style of yoga where postures are held for approximately 3 to 5 minutes to connect to the deep parts of our joints and ligaments. Props are used to support the body in relaxing postures. (While this isn't a traditional form of yoga, I do personally find it helpful as it encourages us to slow down and be mindful.)
- Hot yoga* (modern yoga) – A modern form of yoga located in a sauna-like environment, which is aimed at helping with weight loss. Hot yoga mainly concentrates on the physical side of yoga and emphasises flexibility. It doesn't often dive into the spiritual aspects found in traditional yoga practices. This form of yoga originated with Bikram Yoga, which has been renamed due to recent controversies.
- **Iyengar** yoga (modern yoga) – The focus in these classes is on alignment in postures. The use of props is greatly encouraged to achieve proper alignment.

Types of traditional yoga:

- **Haṭha** yoga (traditional yoga) – This doesn't only mean **āsana** (as so many people believe!). Instead, **Haṭha** yoga provides us with practices that help us to cleanse our internal bodies in preparation for deep spiritual practices.
- **Aṣṭāṅga** yoga† (traditional yoga) – A system aimed at achieving spiritual liberation as taught by Sage Patañjali. This system consists of eight limbs that are designed to guide practitioners towards self-realisation and inner peace.

* Hot yoga: Historically, ascetics practised something similar to hot yoga called **panchagni tapas**, an intensive discipline. However, it's not something most people should attempt unless they have immersed themselves deeply in asceticism or traditional yoga culture.

† **Aṣṭāṅga vinyāsa:** You may have heard of the modern-day **Aṣṭāṅga Vinyāsa**, which is a series of **āsana** practices linked with breath (**vinyāsa**) that are widely practised in the modern day and that were popularised by Śri K. Pattabhi Jois. However, this is not to be confused with the traditional style of **Aṣṭāṅga** that we will be discussing; **Aṣṭāṅga** as systematised by Sage Patañjali in the form of **Rāja** yoga and the eight limbs.

- **Kriyā** yoga (traditional yoga) – This style of yoga is often associated with the teachings of Paramahansa Yogananda (discussed on p. 98) as he introduced it to the Western world in his book *Autobiography of a Yogi.* **Kriyā** yoga focuses on purifying the mind through a combination of breathing exercises, meditations and ethical principles. It involves developing a regular meditation practice that will ultimately lead to inner awakening and spiritual growth.
- **Yoga Nidrā** (traditional yoga) – A relaxation technique used to cultivate a deep state of inner stillness and awareness. **Yoga Nidrā** is a kind of guided meditation that leads practitioners into a deep state of relaxation while remaining conscious.

Seeing the list of modern and traditional yoga styles side by side demonstrates how easy it would be for anyone new to the practice to find it impossible to distinguish between them! But one immediate and easy way to add authenticity to your current practice is to use this list to begin choosing classes that align with traditional yoga rather than the modern styles.

A moment of introspection

Now that we have covered the three key teachings and the styles of yoga, let's take a moment to think about what we've learned.

- Did you know about any styles of yoga beforehand?
- Are there any that you're curious to learn more about now?
- How do you think understanding the differences between modern and traditional yoga styles could change your own yoga journey?

3

Traditional yoga: the four key mārgas

According to the *Bhagavad Gita* (see p. 87), there are four key **mārgas*** (or classical paths of yoga, as they're also known) to attain **mokṣa** (liberation). One of our great gurus, Swami Vivekananda, extracted these four paths of yoga from the *Bhagavad Gita*, simplified them, and compartmentalised them into four key concepts of yoga for different personality types.†

Although all four **mārgas** are believed to align with different personalities and temperaments, and each has its own unique intention and focus, the goal for practising the **mārgas** remains the same: for a practitioner to incorporate elements from all four paths into their practice to help balance their mind and emotions. The purpose of these **mārgas** is to reduce ego and attachment, paving the way for self-realisation and **mokṣa**.

These **mārgas** can act as a great foundation for your practice, and they're also the most accessible way of practising yoga. This is because the paths are mostly based on spiritual practices rather than practical exercises, so your practice is not limited by what your body can physically do. In this chapter, we'll explore each of these four **mārgas** in turn. They are:

1. **Karma** yoga - The path of duty and service.
2. **Bhakti** yoga - The path of devotion.
3. **Rāja** yoga - The path of self-realisation.
4. **Jñāna**‡ yoga - The path of knowledge and wisdom.

* **Mārga:** The term **mārga** translates to 'path', and it's worth noting that **mārga** refers to a spiritual path. This is different from the various 'styles' or 'types' of yoga mentioned in previous chapters, such as **Haṭha**, **Vinyāsa** and **Iyengar**. These types or styles of yoga were developed more recently. In contrast, the **mārgas** are from the Vedic era (see p. 75) and are spiritual paths to yoga organised by personality type.

† There are 18 types of yoga (including **Kriyā** and **Mantra**) that can be interpreted from the teachings of the *Gita*. While all these types are not explicitly named in the text, the wisdom and insights of the *Gita* still offer valuable understanding about them.

‡ **Jñāna** is pronounced as 'nyah-nuh', The 'J' is pronounced as 'ny'.

Nowadays, it's common for people to categorise themselves into one group. For example, certain people may identify themselves as being a '**Bhakti** yogi' or a '**Rāja** yogi'. Each **mārga** has a specific focus but you will notice some similarities between them all. It's therefore important to understand that these paths can be used interchangeably based on your personal preferences and goals. When any of the paths are followed with complete devotion, it's inevitable that you will become familiar with all the others along the way.

I'll be explaining each **mārga** to you, so I recommend reading through them all first to see which ones align with you best. As we go through, you may find that only one or two paths resonate with you, and that's perfectly fine. If all four resonate, that's brilliant, but remember to take it one step at a time.

A couple of points before we get started:

- First, the following **mārgas** are in line with what the *Bhagavad Gita* teaches us. They should be performed while focusing either on the intention of the spiritual goal of **mokṣa** OR while focusing on your own personal spiritual goal. Without this intention in mind, the focus is drawn to external actions, which defeats the point of the practices.
- Second, the **mārgas** are intertwined with **Sāṃkhya** philosophy (one of the six schools of philosophy taught in Hinduism). As we learned on p. 112, yoga as a concept is based on the practical implementation of **Sāṃkhya**, which believes the path to liberation is through self-realisation. Therefore, the practices I will be sharing in this chapter will give you greater insight into the **Sāṃkhya** school of thought and will be focused on self-realisation.

It's time to meet the **mārgas**. We'll go through each one in turn.

Mārga one: Karma yoga

A lot of people link the term **karma** with 'what goes around, comes around'. Although partially true, this is a very bland interpretation of the word and doesn't capture the full depth of its meaning, so let's expand on it.

The term **karma** is a yogic concept and, in this context of yoga, it is a means of action or work that purifies the mind and encourages *selfless* action. A '**Karma** yogi' gives without any desire to receive or to gain any benefit for themselves, and they practise with the purest intentions.

Practising **Karma** yoga, according to yogic texts, is said to purify and expand the heart while destroying the barriers that prevent us from achieving unity or oneness.

Here's where 'what goes around, comes around' comes in: within yogic philosophy, we are taught that each cycle of **saṃsāra** (the cycle of birth, death and rebirth, p. 79) consists of accumulated **karma** based on our actions in our last life. This **karma** is based on our thoughts, intentions and actions, and our **karma** influences the quality of our next life. During each lifetime we can accumulate **puṇyā** (positive/good **karma**) or **pāpa** (negative/bad **karma**). Practising **Karma** yoga helps us in breaking free from **saṃsāra** so that we can reach **mokṣa**.

Chapter three of the *Bhagavad Gita* teaches us about the importance of **Karma** yoga when Lord Krishna describes two paths that lead to enlightenment:

1. Knowledge based on **Sāṃkhya**
2. Action or work

Let's unpack both of these.

First, the *Gita* teaches that investing in understanding and applying the knowledge that is taught in **Sāṃkhya** philosophy is one way of managing our actions and their effects (**karma**) – which we will be doing a lot of in this book!

Second, it shows that **karma** also happens when you take actions or carry out work duties selflessly *without* attachment to the action itself and without attachment to the personal gratifications of the action or work, whether it be for yourself or for others. When we practise **Karma** yoga in this way, we become more aligned with **sāttvic*** choices and actions. For instance, as a schoolteacher, it's important not to show favouritism towards one child simply because you have a personal preference for them. This would indicate a bias towards an outcome that benefits you. Another example is helping at a homeless shelter and filming it purely for the intention of gaining likes on social media. This is acting for personal reward and doesn't align with the values of **karma**.

* **Sāttvic** means 'purity', and in this context **sāttvic** choices are decisions that are made from a calm and balanced state. Cultivating mental clarity through a **sāttvic** mindset ensures that we are operating from a place of harmony rather than fear.

Karma yoga teaches us to perform actions with a selfless and compassionate heart. Practising in this way helps us to develop humility, empathy and connection to those around us, and ultimately brings us closer to liberation.

Did you know?

Interestingly, a study carried out in 2013 on the effects of **Karma** yoga on positive psychology and well-being found that it can be used as a therapeutic method for reducing anxiety and stress.

This short quote from the *Gita* sums up **Karma** yoga:

तस्मादसक्त: सततं कार्यं कर्म समाचर |
असक्तो ह्याचरन्कर्म परमाप्नोति पूरुष: || 19||

tasmād asaktaḥ satataṁ kāryaṁ karma samāchara
asakto hyācharan karma param āpnoti pūruṣhaḥ

'Therefore, without attachment, do thou always perform action which should be done; for, by performing action without attachment man reaches the Supreme.'

– *Bhagavad Gita* (3:19) by Swami Sivananda

Essentially what Lord Krishna is saying here is that in order to reach the highest form of **mokṣa** we should perform all actions without an attachment to the outcome. When we are tied to the outcome, we bind ourselves to the cause of **saṃsāra**.

The practice of **karma** can show up in many ways in our lives. Let's look at three ways that you can practise **Karma** yoga.

Three ways that you can practise Karma yoga

1. RELEASING ANY EGO THAT MIGHT BE ATTACHED TO THE RESULT OF ACTIONS

To do this we must try to only do good deeds that aren't motivated or driven by rewards. Thinking of what you might gain from your actions takes away from learning to act selflessly, and acting selflessly is what

Karma yoga teaches. Once you detach from the fruits of your actions then your ego is eliminated, and the heart is purified. **Vairāgya** is a Sanskrit term used in Hindu philosophy that means 'to detach', normally from material gain. The need for these personal and material gains is usually caused by sensory pleasures in the body, which we often give in to because of our attachment to the body.

Obviously, no one is perfect and the goal of subsiding the ego and releasing attachment does not come easily. But once you learn to free yourself from this then a state of bliss can be experienced, and your true nature is felt (or your true Self, which brings you closer to conscious awareness).

Examples of how you can release your ego vary from volunteering at your local shelter to helping a neighbour. The important thing here is to have the intention of serving others out of compassion, whether that be by cooking for a good friend or donating blood. Teaching or sharing your skills are also ways of practising **Karma** yoga, as long as these duties are carried out without expecting anything in return.

2. HAVE CLARITY IN YOUR DUTY AND HAVE CONFIDENCE IN THE IMPORTANCE OF YOUR WORK

Finding your **dharma** (duty) or life purpose, and having clarity around what that may be, isn't an easy job. I know that I didn't find mine until my early thirties and it's OK to not know until much later still. Finding this out can be very confusing and it can take a lot of mental and emotional healing before you find it. For example, you may not know whether to leave your job or a partner or whether to change your current living situation to carry out your life duty.

However, once you decide and find clarity in the decision, you can become confident in that decision and surrender to the outcome. When you are confident in the work that you do, you no longer feel a need to be attached to current circumstances or the outcome because you are assured that the result will be positive.

3. WORKING ON LETTING GO OF PEOPLE PLEASING

Putting the needs of others ahead of your own can be a good thing. However, when you do this, you risk losing your sense of Self (your identity) through the need to prove yourself by impressing others.

People pleasing usually means you are seeking validation from another person and therefore have an *expectation of the results from the good deeds you are carrying out* for the said person. People pleasing is a symptom of low self-esteem and often a coping mechanism that stems from childhood to avoid feeling rejected or disliked.

It's worth being aware that people-pleasing behaviour can be a mental health issue, although it's not usually seen as one. People pleasing is a tendency that can develop because of trauma or emotional neglect and can result in feelings of resentment. But one way to practise **Karma** yoga is to perhaps learn to identify this behaviour within yourself, if it exists, and to try to implement changes small or big where you can.

The outcome of practising Karma yoga

Benefits – Practising **Karma** yoga in these ways helps with progression on the spiritual path and maintains **dharma**.* It teaches us how to act in a way that serves the greater good of others with the deepest sense of care.

Effects – It promotes compassion, kindness and joy while reducing negative emotions such as greed, selfishness and envy. It also allows us to embody interconnectedness.

A moment of introspection

Take a moment to think over the questions below:

- Do you feel you have understood the concept of **Karma** yoga beyond 'what goes around, comes around'?
- Can you identify any ways that you already practise **Karma** yoga? If so, how?
- What's one easy way you could integrate **Karma** yoga into your life this week?

* **Dharma** also means recognising and carrying out your duties or responsibilities in different aspects of life to promote personal growth and sustain social harmony.

Mārga two: Bhakti yoga

Bhakti yoga is a practice that has been woven through my family and that was taught to me by my mother and grandfather. It is one of the highest forms of yoga and the essence of yogic philosophy. **Bhakti** yoga is devotional worship or love that is directed towards God (or your interpretation of God) or an **iṣṭadevatā** (personal deity whom you feel most affiliated with). This worship could also be devotion towards a cause, philosophy or teacher. It's where we seek a connection beyond ourselves using our emotions and faith.

Ultimately, it means following something that is **sāttvic** (pure) in nature with awareness and curiosity. That means not blindly following someone or something and, if it happens to be a person, then you would be following their *principles rather than the person themselves*. For instance, if you like my teachings and resonate with the work that I do, then you would follow me for the teachings and not for my personality, my likes and my dislikes. When we get attached or caught up in the person, it hinders our spiritual growth and can often be misleading.

Through practising **Bhakti** yoga, our spirituality and essence of being is reawakened. This frees us from material distress, which can often be the root of our anxiety. Those who implement this practice into everyday life can gradually detach from external or temporary pursuits and become more interested in the **puruṣa** (eternal Self).

This is reflected in the *Bhagavad Gita* as Lord Krishna says the following:

श्रीभगवानुवाच |
मय्यावेश्य मनो ये मां नित्ययुक्ता उपासते |
श्रद्धया परयोपेतास्ते मे युक्ततमा मताः || 2||

śhrī-bhagavān uvācha
mayy āveśhya mano ye māṁ nitya-yuktā upāsate
śhraddhayā parayopetās te me yuktatamā matāḥ

'Those who set their hearts on me and worship me with unfailing devotion and faith are more established in yoga.'

– *Bhagavad Gita* (12:2) by Eknath Easwaran

Lord Krishna is saying here that the greatest yogis are the ones who can find complete devotion for him. Now, you might be thinking this is the complete opposite of what I've just laid out (!) but let me explain. By referring to 'himself' in this context, it's important to bear in mind that Lord Krishna isn't speaking from a place of ego. Full devotion to 'him' doesn't make him superior to anyone (which is why we avoid worshipping an individual). Instead, this reference refers to the concept of keeping a one-pointed focus on whatever higher power you may believe in. Whether that be God, consciousness, spirituality... Whatever it is, you will anchor back to this idol or concept as a way of centring yourself.

Three ways that you can practise Bhakti yoga

1. MANTRA CHANTING ON A DEITY OF YOUR CHOICE

Mantras are sacred phrases, words or sounds that deepen our spiritual experience (as we explored on p. 43). Chanting **mantras** that are specific to the deity of your choice can help to develop a deeper connection to the divine. To concentrate on the **mantra**, you should ensure that you have a calm and quiet space where you can sit upright.

Regular practise of mantra chanting in **Bhakti** yoga can lead to increased spiritual growth and inner peace. Some people also use a **japa māla** (a string of 108 beads) while chanting to help keep track of the repetition of each **mantra**, moving one bead at a time for every time you repeat the **mantra**. If you feel drawn to traditional **mantras** you can explore your response to them. Pay attention to the vibrations and feelings that come up for you while chanting as **mantras** can enhance energy.

2. DHYĀNA (MEDITATION) ON A DEITY OF YOUR CHOICE

First choose the object of your devotion. This deity can be Lord Krishna, Lord Shiva (see p. 89) or any other form of the divine (for example, your inner wisdom or your higher Self). Then find a quiet, clean and sacred space. During this meditation, devotees visualise their deity of choice while being open to receiving any insights or guidance from them. Prayers and gratitude towards their deity are also offered as the practitioner reflects on the qualities of the deity. This practice helps us to cultivate deep spiritual fulfilment and encourages us to have a more intimate relationship with whichever higher divine power we believe in.

3. SETTING UP AN ALTAR WITH AN IMAGE OR STATUE OF YOUR FAVOURITE DEITY AND MAKING DAILY OFFERINGS OF FRUITS, FLOWERS OR INCENSE

The rituals and offerings in **Bhakti** yoga are not about materialistic gains but are a way of expressing our deepest gratitude and devotion to the divine. Deep emphasis is placed on the intention of our offering, which should be made with the most sincerity. Flowers, **agarbatti** (incense), food, **divas** (lamps), water and **bhajans** (chants) are all ways of offering our love to the higher power once we have set up an altar.

The outcome of practising Bhakti yoga

Benefits – There are many ways that we can benefit from the practice of **Bhakti** yoga as it can improve our mental, emotional and spiritual well-being. A regular practice can bring inner peace and reduce stress and anxiety.

Effects – Our minds are more focused when engaging with **Bhakti** practices and our concentration is enhanced. We cultivate gratitude while practising **Bhakti** yoga, therefore reducing negative emotions such as anger or jealousy.

Mārga three: Rāja yoga

Swami Vivekananda describes this **mārga** as 'the real instrument of religious enquiry' where the key parts are: **prāṇāyāma** (breath control), **dhyāna** (meditation) and **dhāraṇā** (concentration of the mind). **Rāja** (pronounced 'Raaj-uh') yoga involves controlling your body, breath and mind so that you can eliminate the ego and reach a state of **samādhi** (bliss). This is usually achieved through meditation and other practices that help to control the mind.

Rāja yoga is **Aṣṭāṅga** yoga, but not the **Aṣṭāṅga** yoga that you might be thinking of from recent times in the Western world, which focuses on physical poses. Instead, I am referring to **Aṣṭāṅga** as the eight limbs of yoga, which are the eight steps that can take us closer to self-realisation. In this sense, these eight limbs focus on disciplining the mind to guide individuals towards spiritual growth. We seldom hear of yogic philosophy in modern classes, and when we do it is normally in the form of describing just one of the eight limbs. I will be going into greater detail about the eight limbs later in **Part 3,** so for now I suggest you simply think of **Rāja** yoga as **Aṣṭāṅga** yoga (the eightfold path).

A lot of the written teachings of **Rāja** yoga were lost in India because of wars and invasions. However, scholars have proven that more than 2500 years ago, Sage Patañjali compiled The *Yoga Sūtras* (which we now know as *The Yoga Sūtras of Patañjali*, see p. 85), where the path of **Rāja** yoga is explained.

The *Gita* doesn't rigidly offer its own chapter to **Rāja** yoga in the same way that it does with the other three **mārgas** of **Karma, Bhakti** and **Jñāna**. However, we can find the practices associated with **Rāja** yoga interwoven throughout the text. For example, in the sixth chapter of the *Gita* there is specific mention of the importance of meditation, as well as other principles that help us to control the mind:

युञ्जन्नेवं सदात्मानं योगी नियतमानसः |
शान्तिं निर्वाणपरमां मत्संस्थामधिगच्छति || 15||

yuñjann evaṁ sadātmānaṁ yogī niyata-mānasaḥ
śhāntiṁ nirvāṇa-paramāṁ mat-sansthām adhigachchhati

> 'With senses and mind constantly controlled through meditation, united with the Self within, an aspirant attains nirvana, the state of abiding joy and peace in me.'
>
> – *Bhagavad Gita* (6:15) by Eknath Easwaran

Lord Krishna is describing here the profound effects of **dhyāna**. He is saying that by constant practice, we can reach high states of bliss and inner peace.

Three ways that you can practise Rāja yoga

1. INCORPORATE AND EMBODY AṢṬĀṄGA YOGA INTO YOUR LIFE

The offerings of **Rāja** yoga encourage us to control our minds using eight steps that guide us closer to the path of self-realisation (otherwise known as **Aṣṭāṅga** yoga). Not only are these steps practised, but they are also refined over and over until enlightenment is reached. This means that an element of self-discipline is required, which is also a key element of this **mārga**. I have offered guidance on how you can begin incorporating these eight steps into your life later on in **Part 3**.

2. BEGIN WITH THE YAMAS AND NIYAMAS (PURIFICATION OF THE MIND THROUGH YOGIC PRINCIPLES)

Rāja yoga also places emphasis on the **yamas** (behaviours, limb one, p. 153) and **niyamas** (self-observations, limb two, p. 158) from the eight principles of **Aṣṭāṅga** yoga. A key part of refining your practice of the eight limbs is observing, understanding and trying to incorporate the **yamas** and **niyamas** into your daily life, so you could begin practising **Rāja** yoga by starting with these two principles. They provide a basis for self-improvement and aid us on our journey of personal growth while making our interactions with others more pleasant. Once you start integrating these principles into your life, you will begin creating a foundation for the rest of your yogic journey.

For example, one of the **yamas**, **ahiṃsā** (often translated as 'non-harming' or 'non-violence') is a principle rooted in the practice of kindness and compassion towards oneself and others, including animals. It entails refraining from causing harm in any form – physical, verbal or emotional. To incorporate **ahiṃsā** into your practice, begin by observing your thoughts during moments of reflection. If any unkind thoughts come up, whether directed towards yourself or others, gently direct your focus by replacing those thoughts with their opposites, cultivating a mindset of kindness and understanding.

3. MEDITATE ON THE WORD OM*

One of the core practices of **Rāja** yoga is meditation. Meditation can appear daunting to many beginners, which often leads them to steer clear of it. But rest assured, I've broken it down for you further later in **Part 3** (see p. 206) but if you'd like to begin incorporating meditation

* **Om** is a mantra or a sacred vibrational sound and holds immense significance in Hinduism. It symbolises Brahman, representing the ultimate reality. Pronounced as 'A-U-M', chanting is also believed to provide us with a direct connection to the divine in vibrational form and links us to divine knowledge. The resonance of **om** is said to enhance **prāṇic** (vital) energy, making prayers more effective. See p. 44 for more.

into your practice right now, I suggest you follow these simple steps to get started:

1. Find a quiet and clean space that's free from distractions.
2. Sit comfortably in an upright position, either cross-legged on the floor or in a chair.
3. Close your eyes or soften your gaze and shift your awareness to your breath.
4. Begin by taking deep inhales and exhales, allowing the abdomen to rise and fall.
5. Now start to introduce the **om mantra** either silently within your mind or by softly saying it aloud. Alternatively, you can play a recording of the **om mantra** in the background, focusing your attention on its significance.
6. Practise for five minutes and then bring your attention back to your surroundings. As you practise regularly, you can gradually increase the duration of your meditation sessions.

The outcome of practising Rāja yoga

Benefits – The regular practise of **Rāja** yoga can help us to cultivate more self-discipline and to develop mental clarity and focus.

Effects – Balanced emotions and stress reduction.

Mārga four: Jñāna yoga

Also known as the 'knowledge of wisdom', this **mārga** takes us on a journey of inner exploration as we're guided to understand the true nature of ourselves. Understanding of this **mārga** comes from **svādhyāya** (self-study) and self-enquiry. When we refer to the term 'knowledge' in **Jñāna** yoga, we are referring to 'knowledge of the Self', where self-discovery and self-awareness lead to enlightenment. This path of yoga is one of the most important for attaining inner peace and contentment with yourself and can help you to transcend through **vijñānamaya koṣa** (a layer of consciousness that represents intellect, wisdom and discernment – see p. 143).

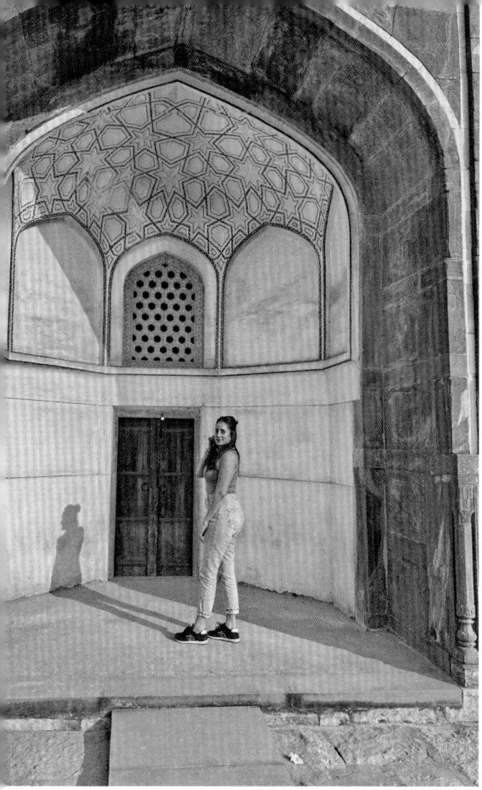

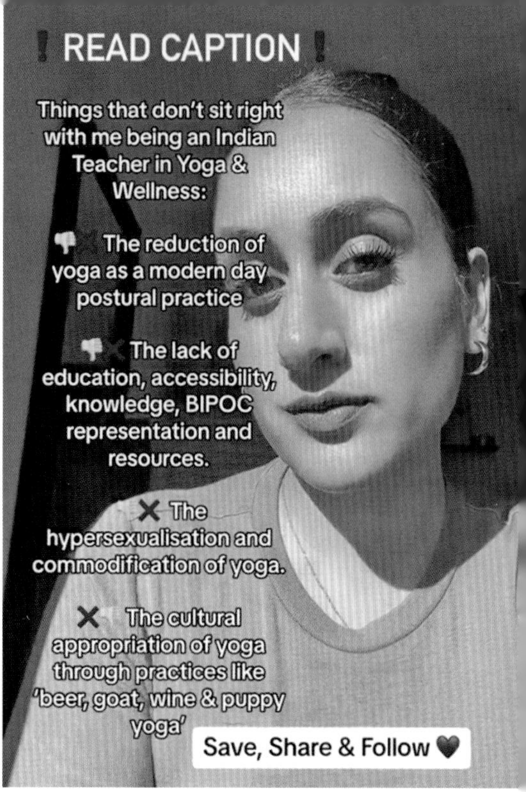

:especting the Indian origins of yoga is key to creating an authentic practice. re I am on a recent visit to India to reconnect with my family's roots.

use my social media to educate people about the issues with Western ga and how to move towards a more respectful practice.

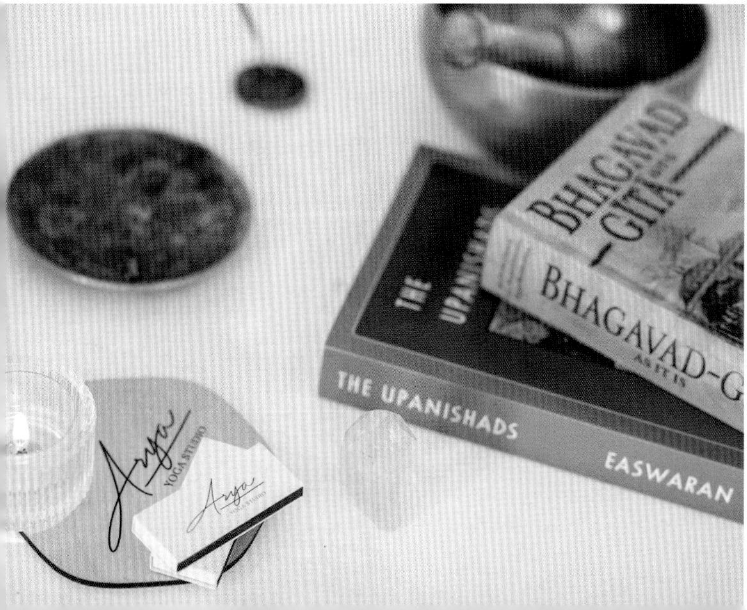

« At my online studio, Arya Yoga, we create a welcoming and inclusive space for our **āsana**, **prāṇāyāma** and self-study practice.

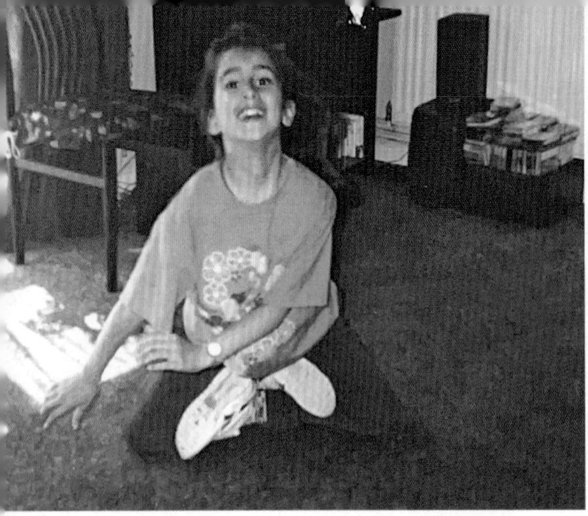

≈ Here I am as a child in an **āsana** (the only one I knew!).

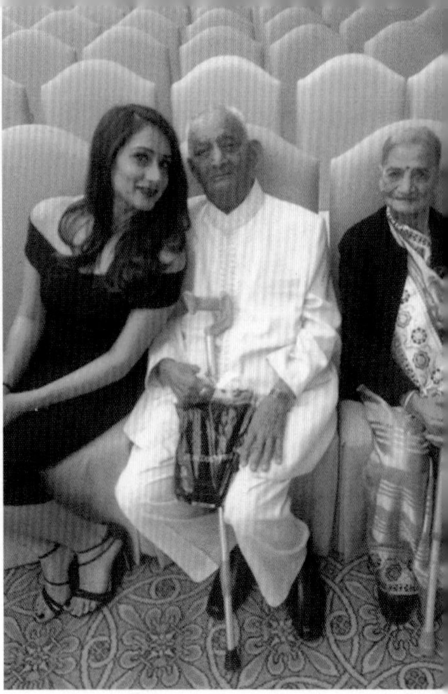

≈ Me with my late grandad and my grandma. They passed down cherished traditions to me, such as writing down sacred **mantras** as a form of meditation.

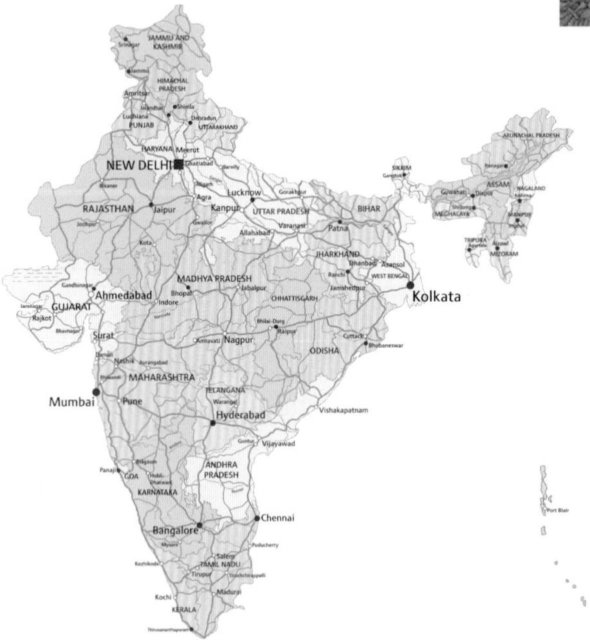

≈ My family are from Gujarat, on the western coast of India.

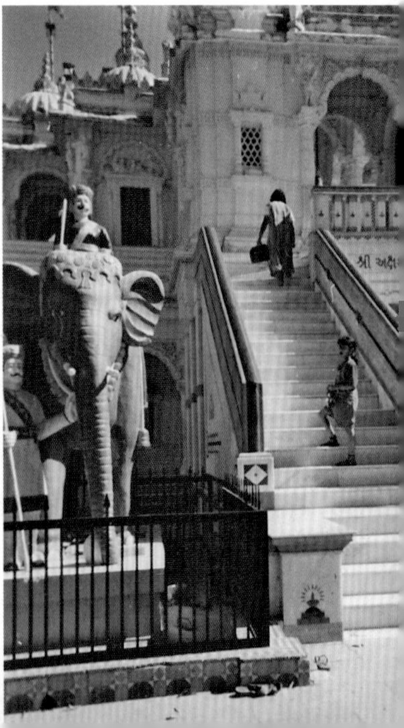

» Visiting family in India as a child – I'm at a **mandir** (temple) in 1996 – helped me to understand my roots and my Hindu heritage.

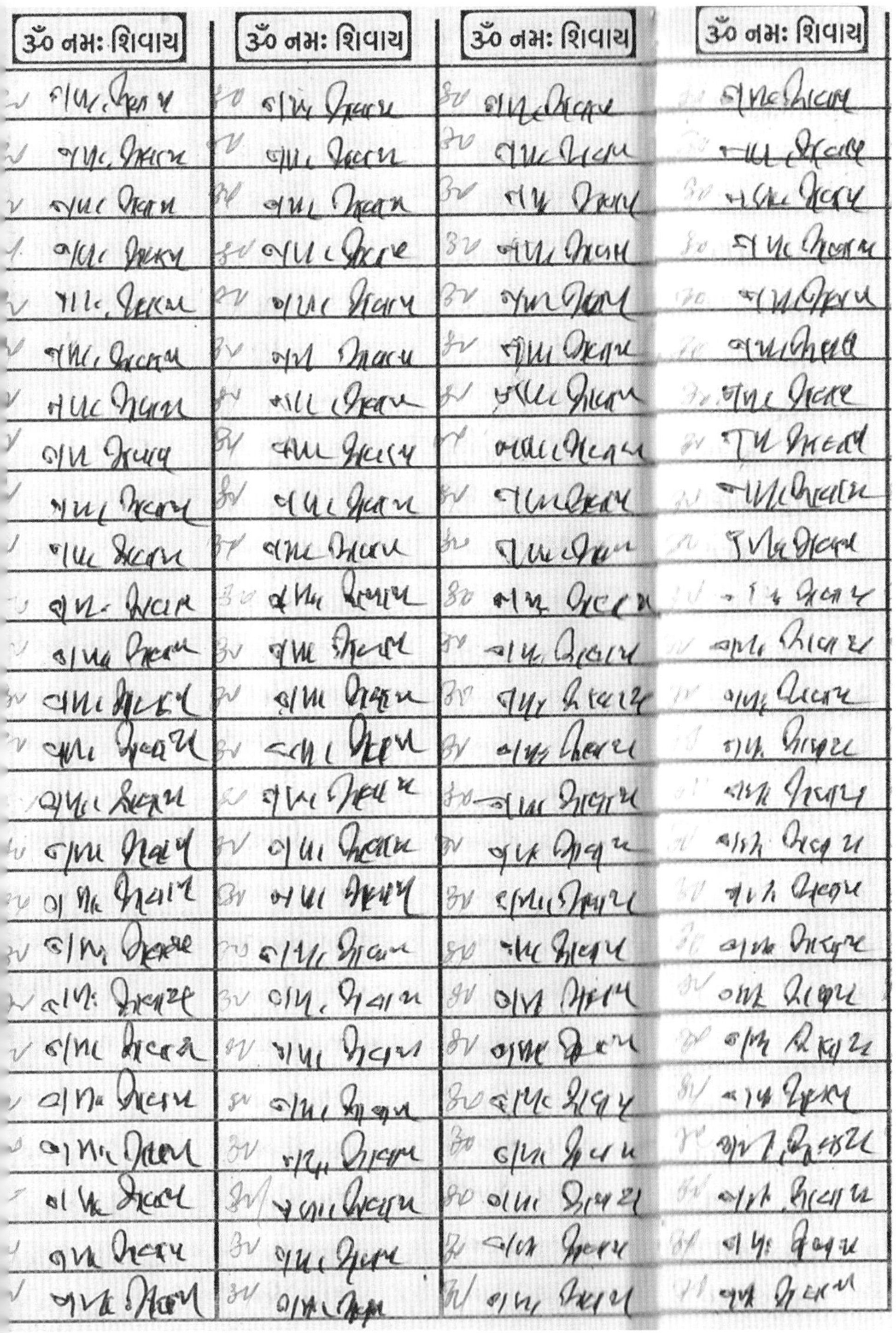

One of many of my grandad's books showing his way of practising yoga aily: by repeatedly writing the mantra **Oṃ Namaḥ Śivāya**, a yoga practice r form of meditation known as **Likhita Japa**.

» Sanskrit script from the *Mahābhārata* – one of the two major Sanskrit epics of ancient India.

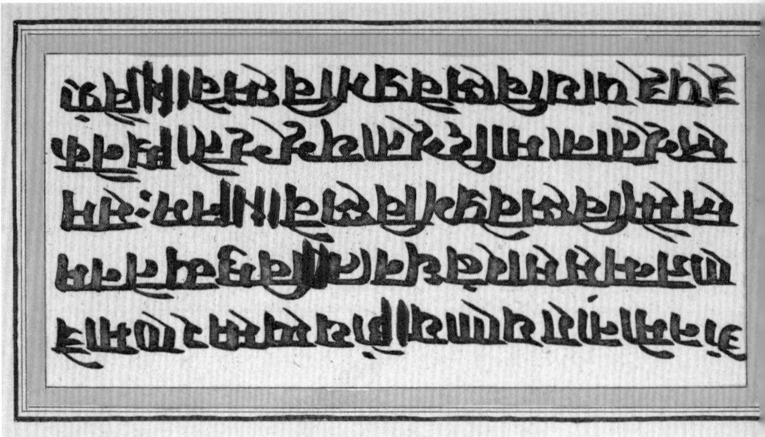

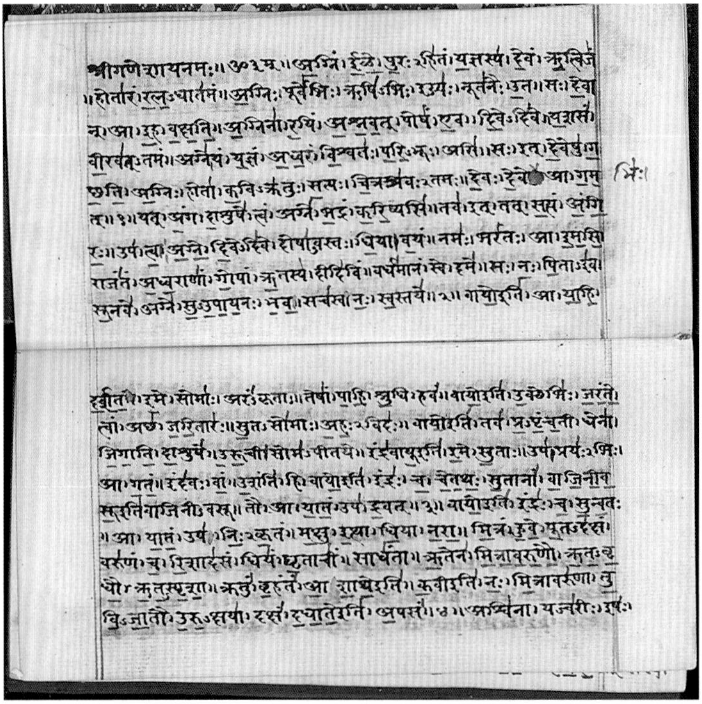

« Pages from **Rig Veda**, the oldest of the four **Vedas**. The **Vedas** are a collectic of ancient Indian hymns that are centr to Hinduism and among the world's earliest religious texts.

» Detail of a preserved palm leaf with writings about **Āyurvedic** medicines in old Malayalam script from Kerala.

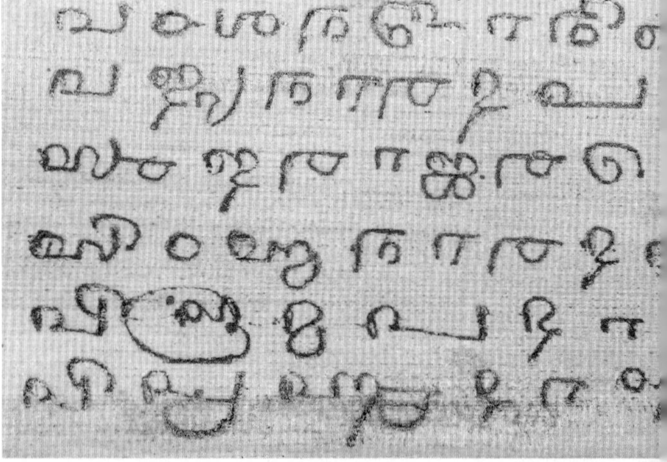

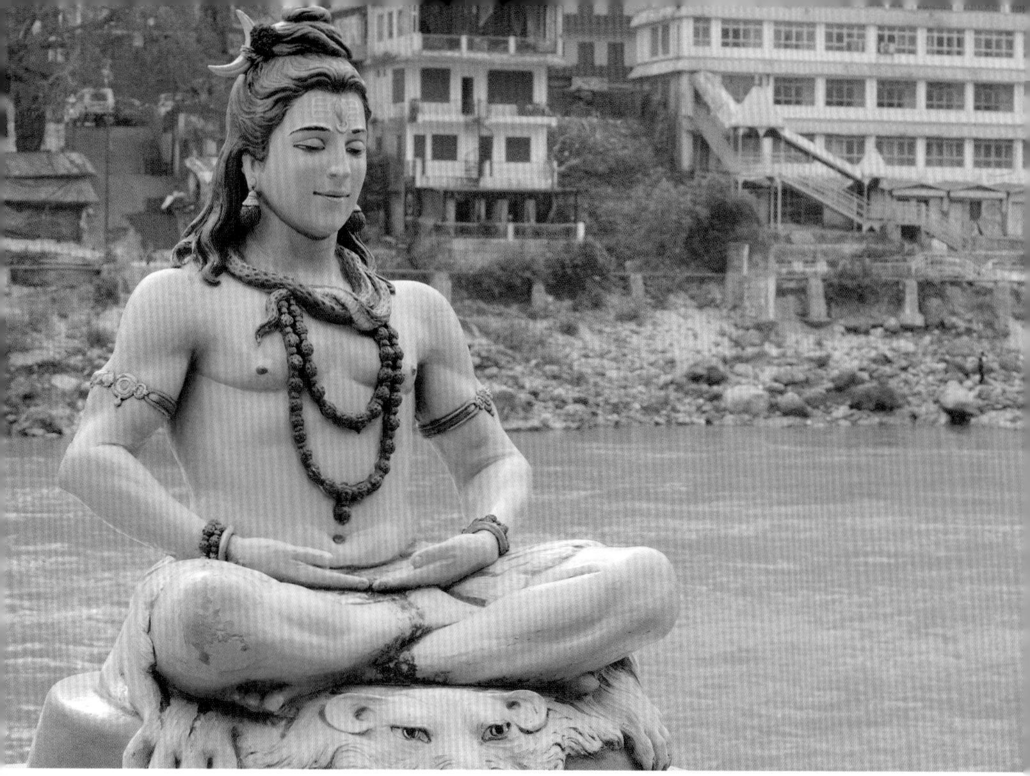

tatue of Lord Shiva in Rishikesh, India. Known as **Adi Yogi** or 'Original Yogi', va symbolises inner transformation through his meditative and disciplined :ure.

tatue of Lord Krishna and Arjuna depicted in a chariot on the battlefield in rukshetra, in a scene from the *Bhagavad Gita.*

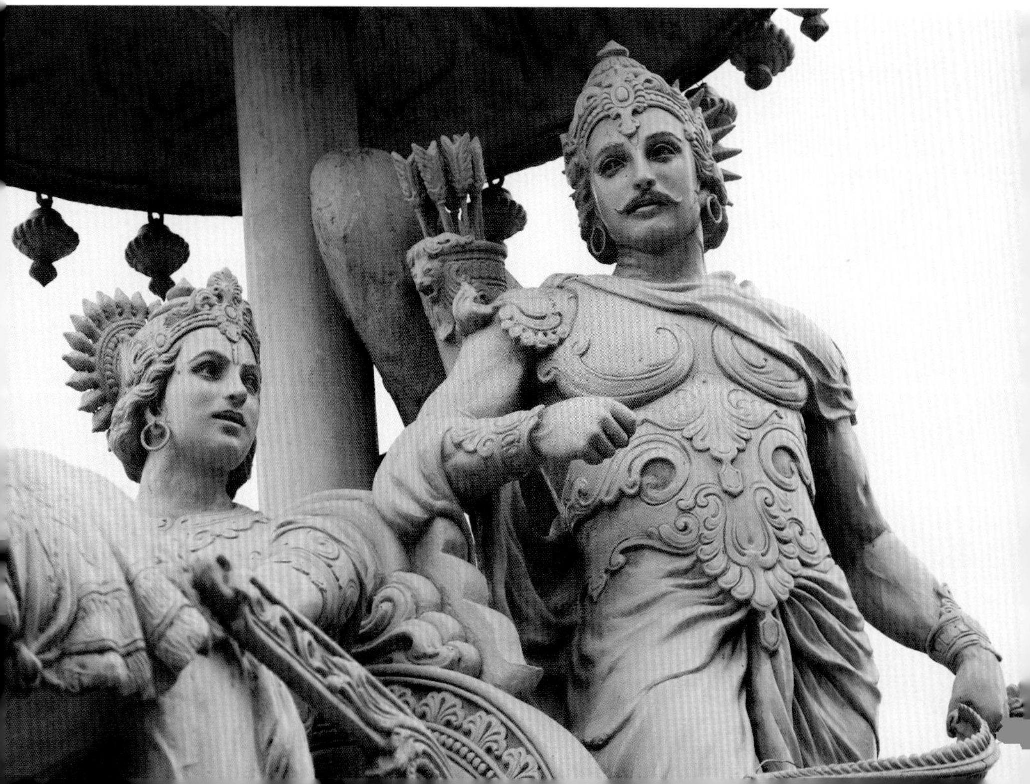

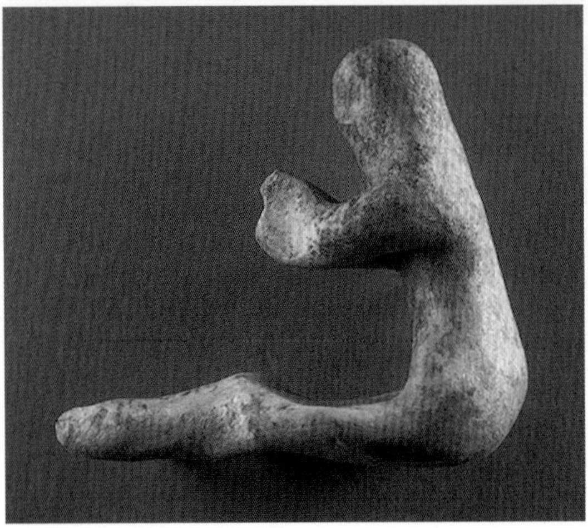

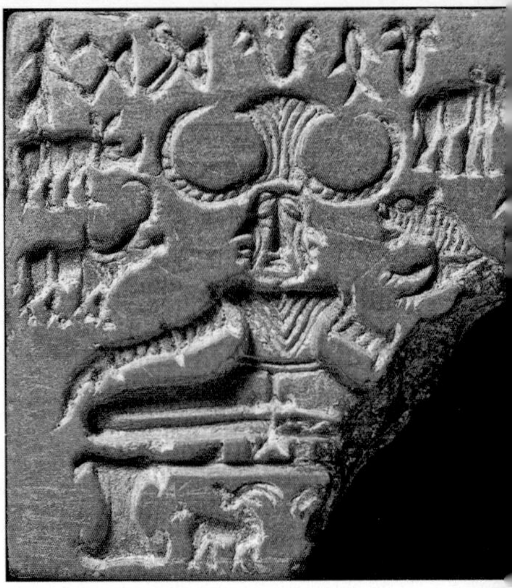

A figurine from the Harappa civilisation. Ancient clay sculptures were found depicting figures in various **āsanas**.

The Paśupati Seal: an ancient artifact from the Indus Valley Civilisation showing a seated figure, often interpreted as an early form of Lord Shiva.

Lord Vishnu, protector of the universe, with Lakshmi at his feet and Brahma on the lotus flower.

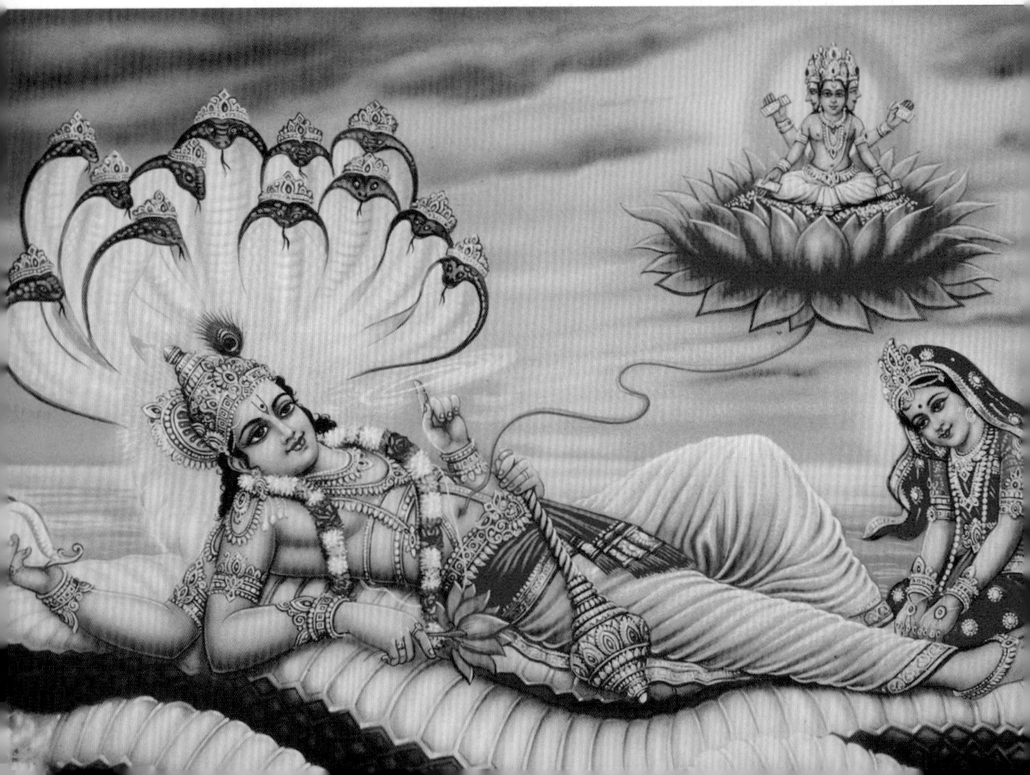

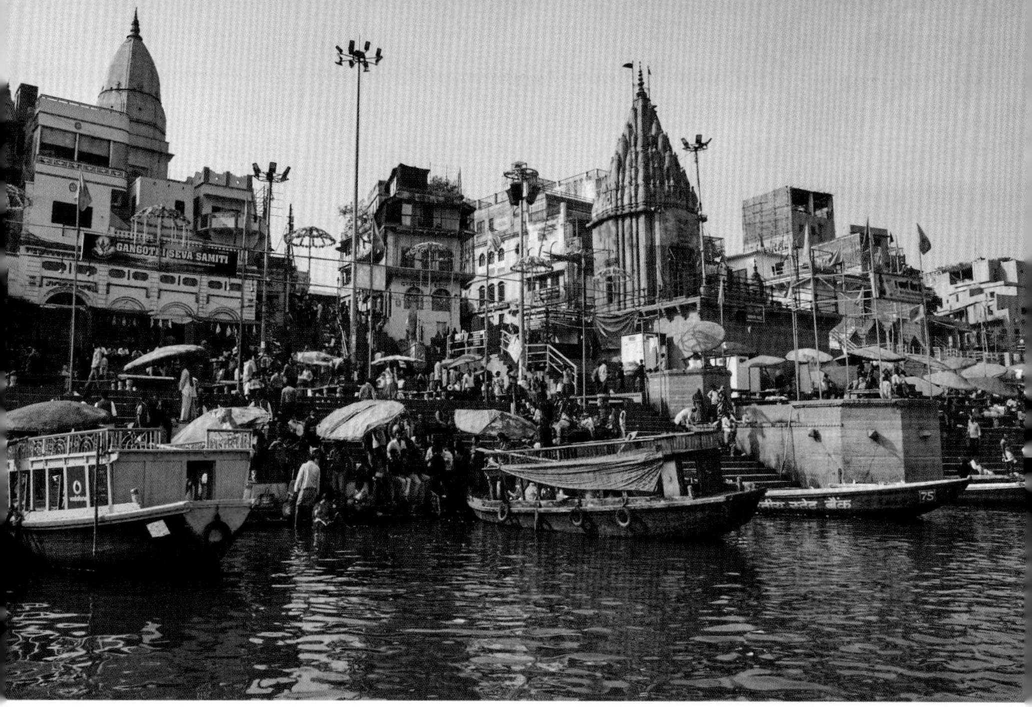

aranasi, one of the holiest ces in India – and a favourite of d Shiva.

wami Vivekananda, an Indian nk who was a key figure in introduction of the Indian losophies of **Vedānta** and ɡa to the western world.

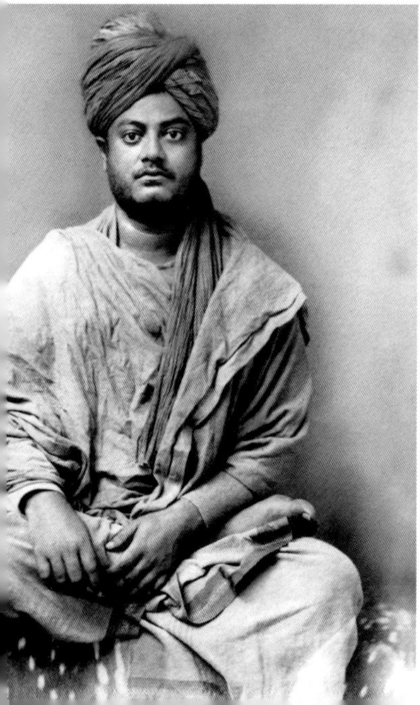

≫ Paramahansa Yogananda, an Indian yogi and guru who introduced many to the teachings of **Kriyā** yoga.

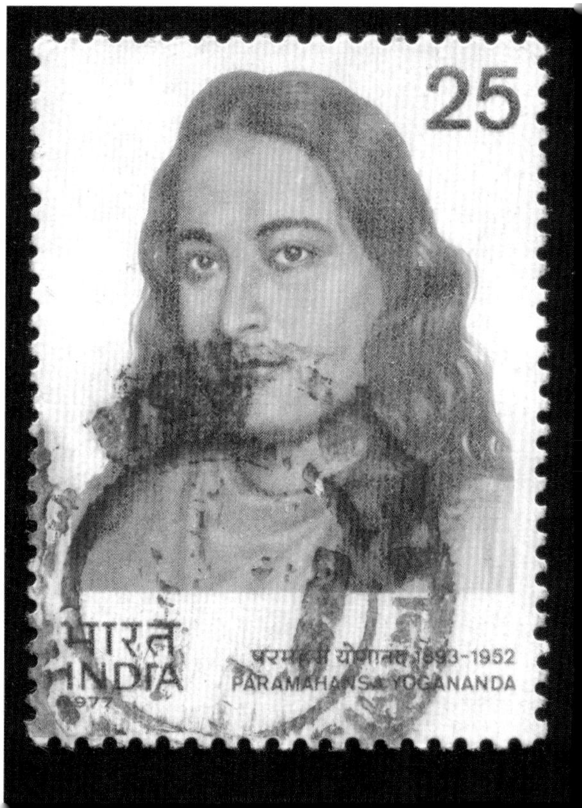

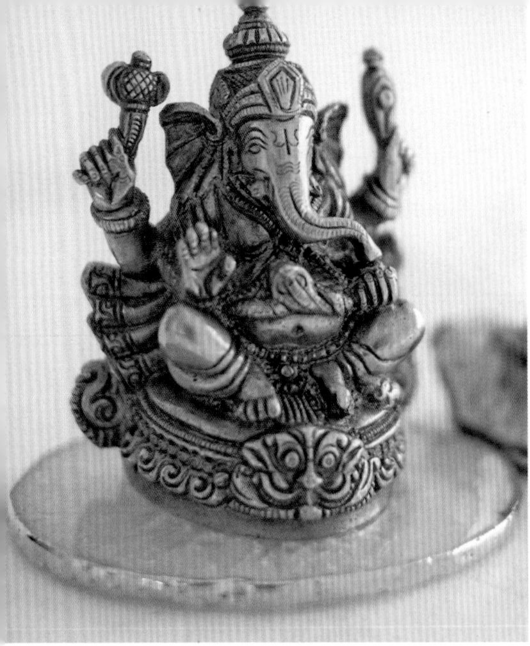

≈ Lord Ganesha is the Hindu deity who is worshipped before beginning any auspicious ceremony.

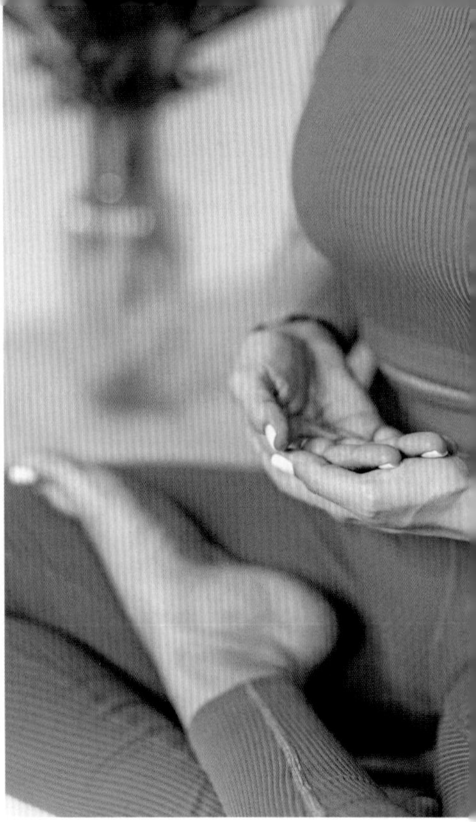

≈ I am demonstrating **bhairava mudra**, which helps channel the flo of **prāṇa** (vital life force energy).

≈ Me in **mālāsana** during my personal **āsana** practice.

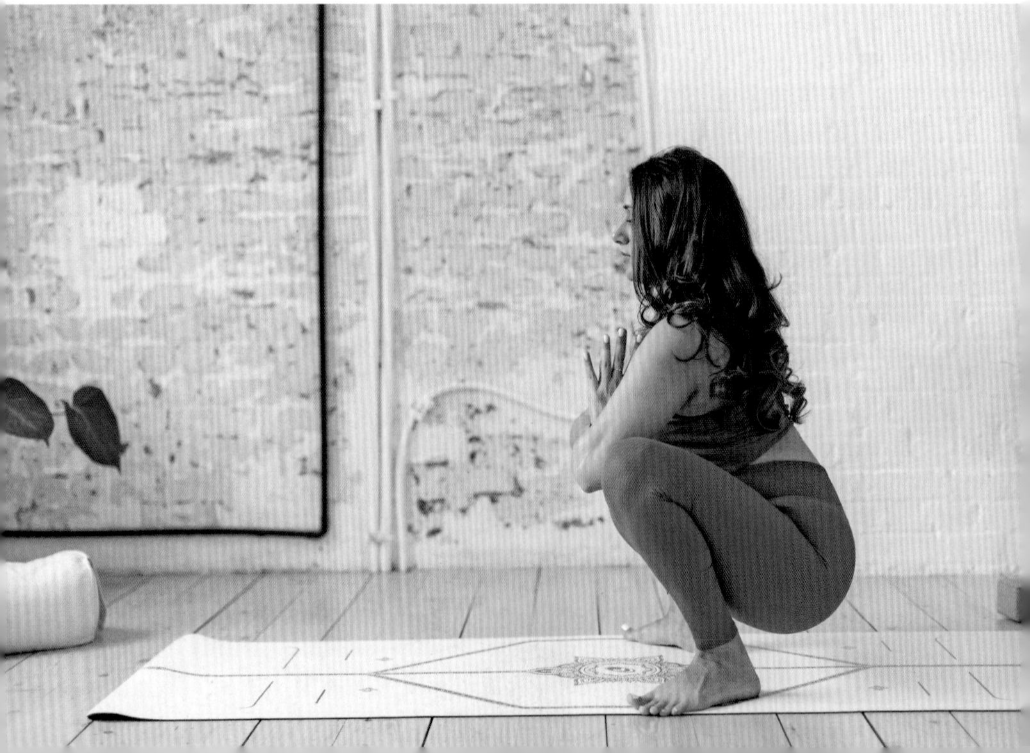

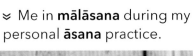

Understanding our true nature is essential for effective implementation of yogic practices. Without this knowledge, navigating the vast world of yoga can feel daunting. Think of it as getting to know your own unique blueprint. By understanding ourselves better, we gain insight into which yogic practices will resonate most with us. After all, if you're not familiar with yourself, it's like trying to find the perfect recipe without knowing your taste preferences.

Just like with **Karma**, **Bhakti** and **Rāja** yoga, **Jñāna** yoga encourages us to detach from the ego. If anything, *more* emphasis is placed on detaching from the ego during this path, as we are aiming to achieve full awareness of the Self.

In the traditional teachings there is an interesting idea that suggests those who practise **Jñāna** yoga embrace a concept of 'gain through losses'. In the context of **Jñāna** yoga, the 'loss' refers to the shedding of one's ego, so in this sense you 'gain' because you have 'lost' your ego. This allows a person to gain through recognising their place as a small part of the vast universe, which enables us to obtain a sense of interconnectedness and appreciate the world around us. In contrast, someone who continuously gathers knowledge in a more traditional sense might gain through feeling a sense of importance and admiration. However, this can sometimes lead to an inflated ego, causing individuals to become overly self-centred and disconnected from the world around them.

Walking the path of **Jñāna** yoga requires an open mind and a curious spirit. If you believe you already possess a wealth of knowledge, it might be a challenge for you to remain receptive to learning more. In a sense, practising **Jñāna** yoga invites us to acknowledge that true wisdom comes from understanding the vastness of what we don't know yet; it's an acknowledgement of the unknown. It can be quite a humbling practice!

Traditionally, **Jñāna** yoga consists of three stages: **śravaṇa** (hearing), **maṇaṇa** (reflection) and **nididhyāsana** (meditation). You can use these as a foundation for your **svādhyāya** when it comes to practising **Jñāna** yoga. Think of them as a framework through which you can gradually expand your practice. For example, **śravaṇa** is the stage of listening to and studying the teachings of wise sages that can be found in spiritual texts or scriptures, so a scripture like the *Bhagavad Gita* would be a great start. Once you have studied the teachings, the stage of **māṇaṇa** encourages us to internalise the concepts and understand the deeper meaning. In the final stage, **nididhyāsana** asks us to become the observer. Here the importance of turning inwards through meditation practices is emphasised.

Let's take my experience of reading the *Bhagavad Gita* and practising **Jñāna** yoga as an example. I knew that reading it once wouldn't be enough to cultivate the self-awareness that I was seeking. Personally, therefore, I've read three different versions of the *Gita* three times, and each reading offered me a completely new perspective. The first time, I was in the stage of listening (**śravaṇa**). During my second reading, I began to internalise the concepts (**māṇaṇa**). By the third reading, I could actively apply these concepts to my meditation practice and experience them more deeply (**nididhyāsana**). This doesn't mean that you must do the same. It simply means trying to dig a bit deeper into self-enquiry every time you have the opportunity to learn something new. That's why **Jñāna yoga** is an integral part of the yogic journey.

Three ways that you can practise Jñāna yoga

1. DEDICATE TIME FOR SELF-STUDY

Using the three stages of **Jñāna** yoga, dedicate 30–60 minutes a week to study a chapter of a yogic text as part of your **svādhyāya**.

For instance, Chapter 2 of the *Bhagavad Gita* is dedicated to **Sāṃkhya** yoga and is where concepts such as the nature of the Self and the importance of detachment are discussed, so you might choose to study this. If you were to use the three stages of **Jñāna** yoga to study this text you could do the following: listen to these teachings with openness (**śravaṇa**), reflect on the importance of these concepts (**māṇaṇa**), and then add these concepts to your meditation practice to find a deeper connection to them (**nididhyāsana**).

Another example would be to study Chapter 6 of the *Bhagavad Gita*, which explores **Dhyāna** yoga. The focus in this chapter is meditation and control for the mind. You can begin by listening to the concepts of meditation and how this helps to discipline the mind (**śravaṇa**), consider the techniques and challenges of meditation (**māṇaṇa**), and then start to engage in a regular mediation practice (**nididhyāsana**).

2. REFLECTION IS KEY

Vichara is a yogic practice that is also a form of self-enquiry or introspection. It encourages us to question and explore our thoughts and ways of thinking so that we can shed the layers of conditioning to discover our true nature. A bit like when people take up therapy or counselling, **Vichara** involves questioning assumptions about yourself, which is why it ties into **Jñāna** yoga. For instance, during therapy sessions, individuals may be asked to question their thoughts, reactions and feelings. But the purpose of the practice of **Vichara** is to go beyond the surface level of your identity, detaching yourself from any labels that you associate yourself with.

To practise **Vichara**, you can try one of the following techniques:

Question yourself

Begin by asking yourself questions about your thoughts, your emotions and anything about yourself generally. Then from here, begin to ask yourself questions that probe deeper inquiry. For example, you might ask yourself 'Who am I?' At this point, don't just take the first response that your mind gives you. Keep probing with follow-up questions like 'Am I x, y, z as a person…?', 'Is this the core of my identity?' or 'Does this profession/career/relationship define me?' Ask another and another question until you gain a deeper understanding of yourself. Begin feeling your answers rather than just thinking of words to label your answers with. This technique encourages deep reflection on yourself.

Picture a scenario

Imagine a situation where you find yourself in a conflict with someone. Instead of dwelling on the disagreement, take a moment to reflect on your actions and behaviours. Ask yourself if you could have made a better effort to understand that person's perspective. Consider how your own actions may have influenced their behaviour or if there is something that you could have done to improve the situation. With practice and patience, this approach can serve as a valuable tool for gaining self-awareness and knowledge of yourself, which is why it's considered a practice of **Jñāna** yoga. Think of it as taking steps to get to know your true Self.

Journalling

Another great way of practising **Vichara** is through journalling, which you can try out as regularly as you can. Journalling is by no means an easy task. If you're not used to writing down your thoughts or feelings, it can prove quite a challenge and it's something I still struggle with at times myself. As a way of beginning, give this short exercise a go:

- Think of a situation that may have brought you feelings of discomfort, anger, frustration or even one where you might have acted out of the ordinary. Take a moment to stay present, gently close your eyes and meditate on it for a brief period of a minute or two. Then write down the situation.
- Next, think about what sparked your thoughts or feelings in that moment. What was the dominant emotion during that situation? How did it make you act or behave? Write it down.
- Finally, close your eyes again and see if you can distance yourself from that feeling or emotion and become the observer instead.

It's important to recognise that releasing an emotion or feeling may not happen instantly. Depending on the circumstances, it could take you several rounds of practising this technique before you notice a gradual shift. The essence of this journalling practice, though, is to raise these questions into your consciousness. This way, the next time (or maybe the time after that) a similar situation arises, your response will likely be altered. Over time, you will be able to navigate through similar situations, increasingly nurturing a greater sense of inner peace.

3. TAKE TIME TO DISCOVER YOUR GURU OR TEACHER

तद्वद्धि प्रणिपातेन परिप्रश्नेन सेवया |
उपदेक्ष्यन्ति ते ज्ञानं ज्ञानिनस्तत्त्वदर्शिनः || 34||

tad viddhi praṇipātena paripraśhnena sevayā
upadekṣhyanti te jñānaṁ jñāninas tattva-darśhinaḥ

> 'Approach those who have realized the purpose of life and question them with reverence and devotion; they will instruct you in this wisdom.'
>
> – *Bhagavad Gita* (4:34) by Eknath Easwaran

Being curious about seeking genuine knowledge from those who are self-realised is essential in **Jñāna** yoga, as they are the ones who will lead you to wisdom and hold you accountable. Someone who is self-realised is usually a guru, so in an ideal world a good way of practising **Jñāna** yoga would be to seek out a guru or authentic teacher (as we discussed on p. 92). Alternatively, if this is not accessible to you, you could begin engaging with the teachings of gurus via yogic literature (p. 94).

The outcome of practising Jñāna yoga

Benefits - **Jñāna** yoga will help to bring clarity to your mind and balance your emotions. It can also be incredibly helpful in shifting your perception of yourself and, in turn, of others.

Effects - A regular practice will lead to a more authentic and purposeful life. The wisdom learned through this practice has a positive impact on our personal growth and spiritual evolution.

The four mārgas – a summary

There is no right or wrong way to practise each of these paths, nor do you need to take on all the practices in one go. These are simply guidelines, and you can work with them and manage them in your own time, at your own pace. Saying that, when you are approaching any of these **mārgas**, remember to practise with *patience* and *consistency*. The more you practise, the more you will see a transformation. Even as a beginner, using these as a foundation for your yoga journey is very valid and over time you will notice lasting changes.

A moment of introspection

The four **mārgas** can be interpreted and used in many different ways. Considering the options that we've talked about:

- Which one or two practices do you think would fit well into your current yoga routine?

Book resources for the four mārgas

Easwaran, Eknath, *Bhagavad Gita* (Nilgiri Press, 2007)
Vivekananda, Swami, *Raja Yoga* (Advaita Ashrama, 2017)
Vivekananda, Swami, *Karma Yoga: The Yoga of Action* (independently published, 2020)
Vivekananda, Swami, *Jnana Yoga: The Yoga of Knowledge* (Vedānta Press, 1998)
Vivekananda, Swami, *Bhakti Yoga: The Yoga of Love and Devotion* (Advaita Ashrama, 2010)

4

Traditional yoga: Haṭha yoga

'A yogi should have a free and open mind.'
– *Haṭha Yoga Pradīpikā* by Swami Muktibodhananda

Understanding Haṭha yoga

A bit like yoga itself, the style of **Haṭha** yoga (pronounced 'HA-tuh') has become associated mainly with physical postures. So much so that when we search for **Haṭha** yoga classes today, it's very difficult to find a practice in its most traditional form (i.e. a class to go beyond only the physical poses of **Haṭha**). Hopefully, after learning more about **Haṭha**'s true purpose here, you'll find it easier to differentiate between an authentic class and the modern interpretation of **Haṭha** yoga.

Swami Swatmarama compiled the *Haṭha Yoga Pradīpikā* (see p. 86), which is the text on which our understanding of **Haṭha** is based. The **Haṭha** branch of yoga represents the balance of contrasting inner energies of the body and mind. These two energies are **ha**, which signifies **prāṇa** (vital energy in the body) and **ṭha**, which signifies the mind (mental energy). When the two are combined – or balanced – which is the goal in **Haṭha** yoga, it's said that our higher consciousness is awakened.*

But what does this mean in real terms for us? Essentially, **Haṭha** yoga places a strong emphasis on purifying the body to allow us to then engage in deeper spiritual practice. By 'deeper spiritual practice' in this sense we often mean **dhyāna** (meditation). So, in very simple

* Higher consciousness: In yoga, higher consciousness means having a broader awareness and a deep understanding of our true selves, where we've moved beyond ego and attachment. It's like experiencing a profound spiritual awakening.

terms, one can view **Haṭha** yoga as a practice in which we help prepare our body for meditation. Our body is purified so that our mind can be awakened. (This has certainly worked best for me, as I've found I'm able to find more stillness during meditation after carrying out **Haṭha** practices.)

To enable us to prepare our body, **Haṭha** yoga places an emphasis on the nervous system and equips us with practices to restore its balance. Through these, we can harmonise our emotions, develop mental clarity and nurture our overall mental and physical well-being. All of this can help prepare us for finding stillness in meditation.

Practising Haṭha yoga

Haṭha yoga practices include a broad range of techniques, including: **prāṇāyāma** (breath control), **mudrās** (gestures), **āsana** (physical poses), **kriyās** (bodily cleansing techniques) and **bandhas** (internal bodily locks), all of which are vital for body purification. However, to begin our **Haṭha** practice, we always start with **āsana** (physical poses) and **prāṇāyāma** (breath control), and we only move on to the other practices once we have familiarised ourselves with both of these. (The fact that **Haṭha** yoga begins with physical poses could be the reason why there is confusion in the West, with some people believing **Haṭha** is only about physical poses because they seldom progress to the other stages.)

Typically, it's recommended to undertake **Haṭha** yoga under the guidance of an experienced teacher, so one way to get started is by attending an authentic **Haṭha** yoga class. However, at the end of this chapter I will also be giving you some simple ways you can start practising **Haṭha** yoga safely as a beginner (remember, even just trying out a few of these practices can have a noticeable impact!).

Before I give you specific practices though, let's talk a little more about the ideal environment to create if you choose to practise **Haṭha** yoga at home, and what you can expect if you choose to practise **Haṭha** yoga in a class.

Haṭha yoga at home – how to create the right environment

I know from personal experience that getting the environment right for your yoga practice can be difficult, especially if you are practising at home. I'm sharing with you now the 'rules' of traditional **Haṭha** yoga, but I suggest you don't stick too rigidly to these. Instead, more realistically, you can simply use them as guidelines to help you establish the most peaceful environment possible while practising. Remember, the mind likes to find excuses to become distracted (as we discussed, along with the other obstacles, on p. 110), so aiming for the following environment can support you in maintaining concentration during your practice:

1. **A spotless and clean space** – The setting you are practising in should be free of clutter and as clean and minimal as possible. 'Even the daily act of cleaning purifies the mind' – *Haṭha Yoga Pradīpikā* by Swami Muktibodhananda
2. **Well-ventilated and quiet** – A space free of pollution where the air is fresh, and the body can remain at a steady temperature. Music is not recommended in traditional practice as it defeats the point of focusing our attention inwards. But, if it's needed to drown out outside distractions, soft instrumental music is totally fine.
3. **No phones** – For obvious reasons! But if you're using one for a YouTube practice, ensure it's in 'do not disturb mode'.
4. **Practising in the same space** – Where possible it is advised, according to the *Haṭha Yoga Pradīpikā*, 'to build up spiritual vibrations'. Whenever I have consistently practised in the same space, I have had people later walk in and say how calming and peaceful the environment is. So, I do believe this holds some truth!

Haṭha yoga in a class – what you can expect

In a traditional **Haṭha** yoga class you'll find a lot of emphasis on **āsana**, or physical postures, because that's where the journey begins. Starting with **āsana** is perfectly fine, especially if you're new to **Haṭha** yoga. It helps you build a solid foundation and makes your practice feel authentic. Once you feel comfortable with the postures, you can gradually explore other cleansing techniques that **Haṭha** offers.

If you decide to attend a **Haṭha** yoga class, then you can expect the following:

1. **Warm-up āsanas** – The first part of the class will involve practising warm-up **āsanas**, which are usually seated postures.
2. **Dynamic āsanas** – Expect 12–15 **āsanas** that will be held for 5 to 10 breaths each.
3. **Prāṇāyāma** – Breathing techniques are carried out after **āsanas** have been practised. During a more advanced class, you can even expect **shatkarmas** (purifying bodily practices) to be incorporated, such as **nauli kriyā** (abdominal massage).
4. **Śavāsana** – Final deep relaxation for 7 to 10 mins.

Naulī kriyā (also known as lauliki kriyā)

Naulī kriyā is by no means a beginner practice. However, since it has gained such popularity in modern-day health and wellness spaces, I thought it would be worth mentioning. (You may have come across this as 'stomach vacuuming'.) I want to touch on this practice mainly as a warning to avoid it (as a beginner), but it's also another good example of how we have seen practices in yoga straying from their origins. Let me explain.

Kriyās are mentioned in **Haṭha** yoga and their purpose is to purify the body physically and internally. According to **Haṭha** yoga, ill health is caused by impurities in the body – physically, mentally, emotionally and spiritually. **Naulī kriyā** or **lauliki kriyā** is a unique method where the internal organs are massaged to stimulate digestion. This is carried out by drawing in the abdomen and rotating the abdominal organs. Sounds complicated, I know! The purpose of this technique is to help to eliminate toxins from the digestive tract.

There are other benefits, too, as it can balance the hormones, purify the nervous system and reduce symptoms of depression. However, in the wellness space, it has gained much attention due to another benefit: the practice can tone and strengthen the abdominal muscles. It has received much attention for this, but the technique can be difficult for beginners to learn, and it requires regular practice before it can be mastered.

→

Naulī kriyā for beginners must be carried out in stages and should be taught with the guidance of a guru or teacher. It should also not be practised during pregnancy or if you experience any health conditions such as hernia, heart disease, gastric or abdominal conditions, or if you are recovering from surgery.

Three ways to begin Haṭha yoga

I won't be able to take you through an entire **Haṭha** class here, but I can give you a few ways of applying some of the teachings, so that you can familiarise yourself with this style and see if it's something you'd like to pursue further. Also, if any of the three practices I share with you here appeal to you, you can include them in your yoga straightaway as an excellent way of immediately enriching your current practice.

1. Āsana (postures)

> 'Being the first accessory of Haṭha yoga, āsana is described first. It should be practised for gaining steady posture, health, and lightness of the body.'
>
> – *Haṭha Yoga Pradīpikā* by Swami Swatmarama

Traditional **Haṭha** yoga involves holding postures for longer durations so that practitioners can fully experience the benefits of each pose. For example, instead of holding a pose for 5 breaths, you hold for 10 breaths. When **āsana** is practised in this way, the mind remains steady and controlled. **Haṭha** yogis believe this approach to be more beneficial for the mind and body.

In **Haṭha** yoga, the **āsanas** suggested are specifically chosen to stimulate the internal organs, energy channels and psychic centres. Some of the **āsanas** that are typically practised during a **Haṭha** yoga class are listed below. You could try including some of these poses into your current practice:

- **Dhanurāsana** (Bow Pose)
- **Paścimottānāsana** (Seated Forward Fold)
- **Padmāsana** (Lotus Pose)
- **Swastikāsana** (Auspicious Pose)

2. Diet

> 'When the body is overloaded with food, it becomes sluggish, and the mind becomes dull'
>
> – *Haṭha Yoga Pradīpikā* by Swami Muktibodhananda

Traditionally, and according to texts like the *Haṭha Yoga Pradīpikā*, a balanced diet plays a key role when it comes to **Haṭha** yoga.

Please note

- What I am sharing with you here is not an attempt to provide you with a dietary plan or nutritional recommendations. The purpose of me including this information is to demonstrate an alternative way of implementing traditional yogic practices, beyond **āsana**. Think about when a personal trainer offers nutritional advice; similarly, yogic culture offers advice on how to maintain a balanced diet, too.
- Different bodies require different diets. Experimenting and finding what works for your body specifically is so important. It's great to explore the traditions of yoga, but remember we need to adapt everything to how we live today.
- Most ancient yogic texts suggest diets that were most suitable for warm or hot climates (i.e. for individuals living in India). You should adapt your dietary requirements to your environment.

As with every aspect of traditional yoga, the teachings should be used as a foundation. There are times when we need to leave room for tweaks or changes.

According to the **Haṭha** yoga tradition, overeating is highlighted as one of the major obstacles that can prove a challenge during our yoga practice.

Haṭha yoga teaches about a diet including:

- Whole grains
- Rice

- Honey
- Dried ginger
- Ghee (clarified butter)
- Brown sugar
- Milk

Of course, this suggestion should be adapted and applied according to your health requirements. However, there may be some foods on the list above that are available to you and that you could think about incorporating as part of your practice if they align with your dietary choices. The texts suggest seeing if you can make a meal using one or more of these ingredients on your days of practising the more physical aspects of yoga, such as **prāṇāyāma** or **āsana**.

3. Prāṇāyāma (breath control)

Prāṇāyāma is more than just breathwork. According to **Haṭha** yogis, once the body is controlled by **āsana** and diet, **prāṇāyāma** can be practised. When **prāṇa** (spiritual energy) accumulates anywhere in the body and becomes stagnant, there is more chance of illnesses occurring. When we use practices like **āsana** and **prāṇāyāma**, we can manipulate the **prāṇa** and encourage it to move freely.

SAMA VRITTI PRĀṆĀYĀMA

A simple **prāṇāyāma** that you could begin with is **Sama Vriti Prāṇāyāma**, or equal breathing. This practice teaches four stages of breathing in which each breath is counted for the same amount of time. It can be practised on its own or alongside an **āsana** practice.

To practise, follow these steps:

1. Sit in a comfortable upright position and rest your hands on your legs with your palms facing up.
2. Close your eyes or soften your gaze and begin to notice the natural rhythm of your breath.
3. Take three deep inhales and exhales.
4. Now begin inhaling through the nose for the count of 4, 3, 2, 1.
5. Hold your breath for 4, 3, 2, 1.

6. Exhale for 4, 3, 2, 1.
7. Hold for 4, 3, 2, 1.
8. After each round, take a moment in silence and stillness to allow your breath to absorb the effects of the practice.
9. Repeat for four rounds and build this up as your practice becomes more regular.

The benefits of this exercise are that it:

- increases lung capacity
- increases mental clarity
- reduces stress and anxiety

A moment of introspection

After exploring **Haṭha** yoga in a bit more depth, let's pause for a moment to reflect on what we've learned and how it resonates with us.

- Have you tried **Haṭha** yoga before? Does it appeal to you?
- What one technique from **Haṭha** yoga could you experiment with incorporating into your current practice?

Book resources for Haṭha yoga

The most authentic practices of **Haṭha** yoga can be found in the *Haṭha Yoga Pradīpikā*. However, this is written in Sanskrit so there are a few translated versions available. Of these, I recommend the following two as the teachings remain the most authentic:

- Muktibodhananda, Swami, *Haṭha Yoga Pradīpikā* (Bihar School of Yoga, India, 1998)
- Swatmarama, Swami (translated by Pancham Sinh), *Haṭha Yoga Pradīpikā* (Pacific Publishing Studio, 2011)

→

Exploring the Subtle Body in Haṭha yoga

In **Haṭha** yoga, we learn that we're made up of three bodies: the Physical Body, the Subtle Body and the Spiritual Body. The Subtle Body, also known as **Sūkṣmaśarīra**, is the part of us that goes beyond what we can see. It's a bit like understanding the deeper layers of yoga that aren't just about physical movements.

Understanding the Subtle Body

1. **Prāṇa** – This is the energy that's connected to our breath, flowing through our body in channels called **nāḍīs**.
2. **Nāḍīs** – Think of these as energy pathways. There are many, but we focus on three main ones: **sushumna**, **iḍā** and **pingalā**. They can influence how energised or calm we feel.
3. **Chakras** – These are energy centres along the spine. They affect our emotions and thoughts, and we can use them for focus during practices like meditation.
4. **Koṣas** – These are like layers of who we are, from our Physical Body to our inner bliss. They help us understand ourselves better.

The five **koṣas** are:

- **Annamaya koṣa** – Our Physical Body is how we interact with the physical world.
- **Prāṇamaya koṣa** – The body of **prāṇa** consists of functions that help keep us alive, such as breathing and digestion.
- **Manomaya koṣa** – Our emotional body where we process our experiences and emotions.
- **Vijñānamaya koṣa** – The body of wisdom and spiritual growth and development.
- **Ānandamaya koṣa** – The body of bliss, where we find inner peace and joy.

Think of the three **koṣas** between the Physical Body (**annamaya koṣa**) and the bliss body (**ānandamaya koṣa**) as the areas we focus on in our yoga practice; breathing, working on our emotions, and enhancing our spiritual development. Working on these helps us move closer to **mokṣa**, or liberation.

→

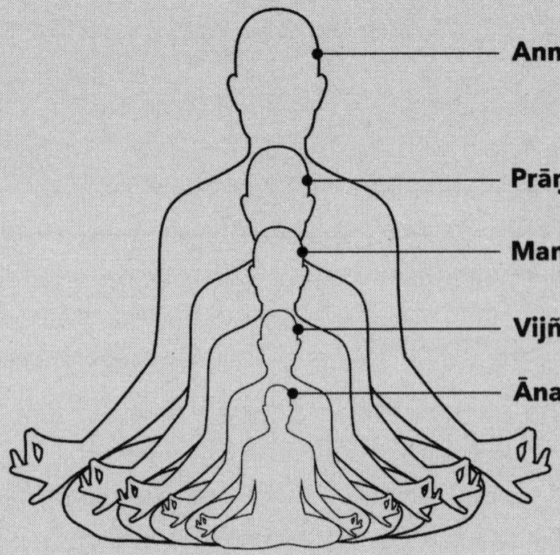

Why it matters

Understanding the Subtle Body in **Haṭha** yoga helps us to see why the practices it offers involve more than just physical poses. Practices like **prāṇāyāma** and **dhyāna** aren't just about relaxation; they're about connecting with our deeper selves for mental and emotional well-being along the path of **Haṭha** yoga.

A note on Āyurveda

Since we have spoken about cleansing the body through **Haṭha** yoga practices and touched on diet in yoga, let me tell you a little more about yoga's sister science: Āyurveda

Āyur = 'life or longevity'
Veda = 'knowledge or science'

Āyurveda is an ancient scientific medical system that was derived in India over 5000 years ago. It encourages nourishment of the mind and body through its classical teachings, treatments and techniques, which restore balance. It therefore holds the same common principles as yoga. As with yoga, this tradition encompasses taking care of mental and physical health. However, in **Āyurveda**, diet is the main focus: the practices suggest making lifestyle adjustments to our diets, using natural remedies and herbal medicines to prevent health issues.

The practice of **Āyurveda** involves using methods that balance our **doṣas** (functional energies) and is thought of as a lifestyle that includes natural therapies. Not only does the age-old science work for the mind and body, but also for the senses, spirit and soul. The system, when applied correctly, also provides us with a holistic approach in treating and curing chronic diseases and illnesses. Although many **Āyurvedic** rituals can take weeks, months or sometimes even years to work, many studies show that the benefits and effects are profound. Many of the methods used are very similar to some of the cleansing practices that we see in yoga. So, both practices can be and *are* usually used synonymously.

Some of the rituals used in an **Āyurvedic** lifestyle to treat imbalances in the mind and body include:

- **Panchakarma** (five actions) – A cleansing method used to detoxify and purify the body internally.
- **Abhyāṅga** – A daily head-to-toe self-massage using herbal-infused warm oils that promote nervous system health.
- **Gandusha** – Oil pulling, which involves holding oil in the mouth for a period of time to promote gut health and prevent diseases of the mouth.
- **Jihwā prakṣālana** – Removing toxins from the body by gently scraping the tongue. This is an ancient practice that has been used for generations and is also said to help improve the digestive system.

These are just a few of many! **Āyurveda**, just like yoga, has an endless number of practices that can improve your overall well-being. It's a practice that is still widely used in India and all over the world and is certainly worth exploring if you are into natural ways of healing.

Book resources for Āyurveda

Charaka, Acharya, *Charaka Samhita: Handbook on Ayurveda* (independently published, 2016)

Lad, Vasant, *The Complete Book of Ayurvedic Home Remedies* (Platkus, 2006)

Bhattacharya, Dr Bhaswati, *Everyday Ayurveda: Daily Habits That Can Change Your Life in a Day* (Random House India, 2019)

5

A note on chakras

Chakras will be familiar to many people within the yoga and wellness space, where they've been interpreted in various ways. While I would not suggest that exploring **chakras** is suitable for beginners in yoga, I think it's important to address them here to clear up the common misunderstandings surrounding them in the West. Similar to terms like **namaste** and **om** (see p. 42), **chakras** have gained immense popularity but are often misinterpreted.

I'll therefore provide a short overview for context here and to clarify their significance, but I won't be including any specific practical practices for you, since traditionally **chakras** are considered advanced. An understanding of **chakras** will help deepen your understanding of traditional yoga, though, and mean you have the correct context if/when you see **chakras** featured in yogic texts or within popular yoga styles, such as **Haṭha**.

What are chakras?

The term **chakra** (pronounced 'chuck-ruh' and not 'sshakra') loosely translates to 'wheel' and, in yogic terms, **chakras** are energy centres that help us to balance the mind and body. There are seven **chakras** that are situated along **sushumna nāḍī** (the central energy channel in our body), and each of these symbolises various aspects of our physical, mental, emotional and spiritual health. Think of each **chakra** as a hub that distributes **prāṇa** (vital energy) to different parts of the body.

Within yoga, the **chakras** are depicted as lotus flowers, each one having a different number of petals. Symbolically, the lotuses all represent three stages of spiritual growth, from the lowest to the highest states of conscious awareness (i.e. being closest to Self).

Each **chakra** is associated with a different colour, and we can also find **yantras** (sacred geometrical images) within each **chakra** corresponding to a different Hindu deity. A dot can be seen on each **chakra** and this is called a **bindu**, which represents our true selves.

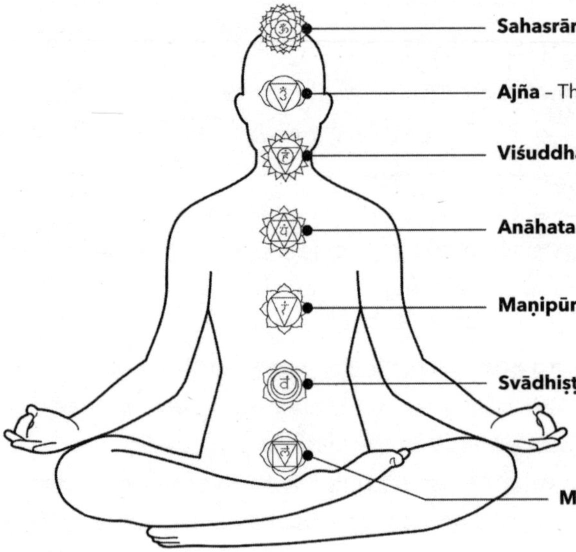

When the **chakras** in our body are balanced, **prāṇa** flows freely through the **nāḍīs** (energy channels) in our body, and we can experience better physical health, emotional stability and spiritual growth. The seven major **chakras**, as indicated on the illustration above, are:

1. **Mūlādhāra** - Root, located at the base of the spine.
2. **Svādhiṣṭhāna** - Sacral, located at the lower abdomen.
3. **Maṇipūra** - Solar plexus, located at the navel.
4. **Anāhata** - Heart, located at the centre of the chest.
5. **Viśuddha** - Throat, located at the throat.
6. **Ajña** - Third Eye, located at the space between the brows.
7. **Sahasrāra** - Crown, located slightly above the head.

Working on **chakras** involves a regular and committed practice, and it's mostly recommended for advanced practitioners. This is because it's important to fully understand and implement practices like **āsana** (physical postures) and **prāṇāyāma** (breath control) before exploring

chakras. If you're keen to work with **chakras** in your practice, I would recommend studying them further by looking at the suggested reading below and in Resources on p. 226.

Book resources for chakras

Muktibodhananda, Swami, *Haṭha Yoga Pradīpikā* (Bihar School of Yoga, India, 1998)

Swami, Om, *Kuṇḍalinī, An Untold Story* (Jaico Publishing House, 2016)

6

Traditional yoga: Aṣṭāṅga yoga

Ashta = 'eight'
Anga = 'limb'

Aṣṭāṅga yoga, aka the eight-limbed path, is a style of yoga that is centred around eight steps (or 'eight limbs') to help us discipline the mind, cultivate inner peace and guide us closer to the path of self-realisation.

Out of all the classical types of yoga, we'll be delving deepest into **Aṣṭāṅga** yoga for two main reasons. First, because **Aṣṭāṅga** yoga is already so common (if often misunderstood) in the Western yoga landscape today, so there will likely be some form of recognition for many readers, which you can use as an entry point to this practice. Second, I've chosen to explore this type of yoga thoroughly because the principles of **Aṣṭāṅga** can be so easily applied to our everyday lives. This means that as we explore the eight limbs of **Aṣṭāṅga** I can offer you many practical examples of how you can incorporate these traditional teachings into your life (and feel the benefits!).

So, what exactly are these eight limbs of yoga? They're used as a practical guide to navigate life's challenges and are rooted in the teachings of *The Yoga Sūtras of Patañjali* (see p. 85), where Sage Patañjali organised them into a system that's easily accessible for everyone to understand. The eight limbs are extremely intricate, though, and can be interpreted in numerous different ways. I've aimed here to simplify them as much as possible to provide an outline for beginners. Here's a summary of the eight limbs to get us started:

1. **Yamas** (our behaviours) – Five ethical principles that make us aware of how we interact with the external world.
2. **Niyamas** (self-observations) – Five personal observances that encourage us to look inwards.

3. **Āsana** (physical postures) – A comfortable seated position or postures that prepare the body so we can sit in meditation for extended periods of time.
4. **Prāṇāyāma** (regulation of breath) – Practices that aid in controlling or regulating the breath.
5. **Pratyāhāra** (influence of senses) – The practice of withdrawing from the five senses and turning your attention inwards.
6. **Dhāraṇā** (concentration of the mind) – Developing focused concentration that prepares us for deep meditation.
7. **Dhyāna** (meditation) – A state of meditation where the mind is quiet and peaceful.
8. **Samādhi** (pure awareness) – A state of complete bliss, enlightenment or contentment.

Each of these limbs allows us to reflect on and examine each aspect of our being. Think of each one as a tool to help us with different aspects of our lives:

1. **Yamas** – social
2. **Niyamas** – personal
3. **Āsana** – physical
4. **Prāṇāyāma** – physiological
5. **Pratyāhāra** – mental
6. **Dhāraṇā** – psychological
7. **Dhyāna** – intellectual
8. **Samādhi** – spiritual

Throughout the following eight chapters, I'll break down the basics of the eight-limbed path, taking each in turn, so you'll have a clear understanding of each limb and how you can integrate the teachings into your daily life.

In what order should I explore the eight-limbed path?

The order in which we approach these eight limbs is specifically designed to guide us from external awareness to internal awareness.

The first five limbs, for example, focus on external (**bāhya)** practices, refining our physical aspects. Then the last three limbs gently lead us inwards, encouraging detachment from the external world as we dive deeper into self-discovery and internal (**ābhyantara)** practice.*

You can certainly switch between the limbs. However, traditionally, and in my own experience, practising them in their intended order does tend to be most beneficial. But whatever order you decide on, the key thing is that you embrace your practice with sincerity and dedication as this is what will ensure you reach your inner state of calm.

Also, I can't possibly cover the full depth of **Aṣṭāṅga** yoga and the eight limbs here. Therefore, I encourage you to take note if any of the limbs particularly appeal to you, so you can continue exploring them further and in more depth through personal study.

A moment of introspection

Before we begin working on our journey of applying the eight limbs to our lives, it is important to acknowledge that we've been shaped by years of conditioning, and we all have our imperfections. This recognition sets the foundation for the self-improvement that awaits us. I invite you to do the following:

- Take a moment to write down your flaws or behaviours that you would like to improve within yourself. Don't be too harsh – remember that the purpose of this practice is to help to make changes for the better.
- Once you have written these down, take a few minutes to notice how those behaviours impact yourself and others. Write this down, too.
- Now let it go and let's continue exploring the path of **Aṣṭāṅga**.

* Different yogic texts categorize the limbs differently. For example,some interpretations of the *Yoga Sūtras* classify the first *four* limbs as external and the final four as internal, but we're focusing on the teachings from *the Yoga Sūtras of Patañjali* here.

7

Limb 1: Yamas (our behaviours)

The first limb within **Aṣṭāṅga** yoga are the **yamas**, which relate to the social aspect of our life.

The **yamas** highlight five behaviours as the practical disciplines required to maintain social harmony between us and the rest of the world. In a sense, they are the principles that teach us how to treat ourselves and others.

The five **yamas** are:

1. **Ahiṃsā** - non-harming
2. **Satya** - honesty or truthfulness
3. **Astēya** - non-stealing
4. **Brahmacharya** - moderation
5. **Aparigraha** - non-possessiveness

Let's look a little closer at each one.

Yama 1 – ahiṃsā

This is commonly translated to 'non-harming' or 'non-violence'. This is the practice of exercising kindness and compassion towards ourselves and others (including animals). It involves not harming anyone or anything physically, verbally or emotionally. The Sanskrit term **hiṃsā** means cruelty or injustice, and **ahiṃsā** is the opposite as it is the practice of not intentionally causing harm to others.

Often, in modern teachings, **ahiṃsā** is portrayed as a saintly virtue where showing a bit of anger gets you cancelled. For example, activists who passionately express their views are frequently labelled as 'angry', even when their anger is justified. However, it's crucial to understand that **ahiṃsā** doesn't suggest that we should never defend ourselves when necessary. Misinterpreting **ahiṃsā** in this way can undermine important voices and messages that need to be heard. Instead, **ahiṃsā** encourages us to be mindful of the potential harm we might cause to others and strive to minimise it. This practice teaches us to cultivate kindness while avoiding harm towards all living beings.

Additionally, it reminds us that we shouldn't rigidly cling to our principles if they prevent us from fulfilling our responsibilities. For instance, if you've committed to volunteering at a charity every Sunday but your grandad needs your help one Sunday because he is unwell, it's perfectly acceptable to prioritise caring for your grandad over your prior commitment to the charity.

To practise

The next time you sit down to reflect, notice any unkind thoughts that might come up regarding yourself or others. Each time one pops up, counteract that thought by thinking the opposite of that person/yourself.

Yama 2 – satya

This is honesty and truthfulness in thoughts, words and actions. It means speaking the truth but not so that it is harmful to others; if the outcome of your truth is going to be negative, don't say it. **Satya** is more than just not lying; it encourages correcting any behaviour that might lead us to become dishonest. For instance, are we really being honest when we say, 'I don't know' or would we be more honest if we were to say, 'I know, but I can't say'?

Practising **satya** guides us in nurturing honesty within our mind, as we remain true to ourselves while also gaining clarity on our intentions. When we try to practise **satya** regularly, we can cultivate deeper and more authentic connections with others. **Satya** can be practised in the form of admitting to your mistakes, or through being honest with yourself and others without passing judgement.

To practise

The next time you have a disagreement with someone, pause and reflect. Observe your reaction and ask yourself, 'Am I telling them everything is

OK just to keep the peace?' Were you being straightforward with that person if they upset you? Are you able to admit where you may have caused harm intentionally or unintentionally?

Yama 3 – astēya

This is the practice of non-stealing, but this goes beyond simply not stealing material objects. When we speak about **astēya**, we also mean not taking advantage of anyone and not cheating anyone. It's about not stealing in terms of thoughts, actions and words, too. This practice of **astēya** can help us in becoming more content, respectful and grateful.

There are also subtle ways that we could steal from others, such as being dishonest, not respecting boundaries, not sharing things you don't use, overindulging or being envious. All of these can be seen as ways of stealing peace of mind from yourself and others. When we cultivate a practice of gratitude, it helps us to become satisfied with what we have so that we don't have the urge to take from others.

To practise

Write down all the things or people you are grateful for and that contribute to you being a healthy, happy person. What are your strengths? Are there any blessings that you feel really grateful for? These could include gestures or acts of kindness from others. Don't limit yourself to just thinking about physical belongings here. However big or small, reflect on and accept everything you have stated you are grateful for. This will help you on your path to inner peace.

Yama 4 – brahmacharya

This is ultimately an act of self-control and moderation. It can be practised by not overindulging in thoughts, TV shows, sexual activities or anything else. The purpose of this practice is to preserve our energy and then use it wisely and responsibly. **Brahmacharya** teaches that when vital energy is conserved for spiritual growth, our self-awareness deepens.

Did you know...?

In ancient times it was believed that sensual desires and actions required too much energy, which could instead be used for spiritual practice. As a result, people often translate this practice to mean celibacy. But **brahmacharya** doesn't mean refraining from sex. According to scriptures, **brahmacharya** can be observed while still being sexually active as long as the act of sex is done at certain times or on certain days. In other words, the act of sex should be done in moderation, as with everything else.

To practise

Observe where your energy is spent on a regular basis. Write it down or speak to someone about it if you feel comfortable. Reflecting on this can help you see where you want to channel your energy consciously. You may realise you spend too much time on social media, for example, so you might decide next week you want to spend an extra hour with your grandparents or an extra hour practising yoga instead.

Yama 5 – aparigraha

This is a practice through which we are encouraged to avoid greed and the accumulation of unnecessary possessions. **Aparigraha** teaches that we should only possess what is truly required, whether that be related to material possessions, thoughts or emotions. Learning to let go rather than hoard or cling to these things allows us to have faith that the universe will always provide us with what we require, whether we possess it or not. (If you're familiar with the law of attraction, we can make a comparison with this as the law of attraction theory also teaches that once you ask for something from the universe, you should have complete faith that you will receive it.)

Aparigraha asks us to let go of attachment so that we can focus on what matters and be free of **duḥkha** (suffering). Think 'less is more'. In yogic philosophy, **duḥkha** often stems from our attachments, i.e. when we cling too tightly to material possessions or to certain outcomes we're hoping for. If we lose something we're attached to or don't have an outcome we want, then it can cause us distress and suffering. Therefore, letting go of attachments is taught here.

To practise

Think about or write down your desires and most valued possessions. Consider what you truly need. Does that possession or desire own you or do you own it? Is there anything you can release yourself from? For example, check if you own a material possession that you rarely use and, if so, could someone else benefit from it more? It's about looking at our possessions and asking if they genuinely serve us or if they could serve someone else better. Observe the feelings that come up. Do you feel fear or resentment? Or are you happy and hopeful? Practising this over time will lead you to greater contentment and inner peace.

8

Limb 2: Niyamas (self-observations)

The second limb are the **niyamas**, which relate to the personal aspect of our life. The **Niyamas** compromise of five disciplines that relate to our internal (personal) world rather than the external one. They refer to the attitudes that we adopt towards ourselves, so you can think of them as self-observations. These are:

1. **Shaucha** - purity or cleanliness
2. **Santoṣa** - contentment
3. **Tapas** - self-discipline
4. **Svādhyāya** - self-study
5. **Īśvarapraṇidhānā** - devotion to the divine

Let's look at each discipline in turn and how we can incorporate these ideas into our own practice.

Niyama 1 – shaucha

This term means keeping things clean and pure internally and externally. This involves the complete purification of our internal and external realities, where we are encouraged to cleanse every aspect of ourselves. This includes eating habits, avoiding harmful substances, maintaining the cleanliness of shared spaces, personal hygiene and removing unnecessary distractions. According to yogic philosophy, keeping our mind, body, thoughts and environment clean and uncluttered brings balance to our mental well-being and physical health.

Traditionally, there are two types of **shaucha**: **bahir shaucha** (external purification) and **antah shaucha** (internal purification). **Bahir shaucha** is the practice of keeping your Physical Body, environment and actions clean and pure. For example, tidying your living space, showering, washing your clothes or engaging in actions that don't cause harm to others. **Antah shaucha** involves the purification of the mind, emotions and inner Self. This could mean working on cultivating positive thoughts, compassion or gratitude, and also engaging in self-improvement practices (a bit like what you're doing right now!).

To practise

Reflect on areas of your life where you may feel unclean. If it's your surroundings, try and dedicate a day to decluttering and clearing out your space. If this is your body, you can try a cleanse or a fast (only if this is right for you). If it's your emotions, try to write them down on paper and get rid of them by burning them (safely) or throwing them away. To cleanse your internal body, try practices like **āsana** (physical poses) or **prāṇāyāma** (breath control) - you can use the ones in this book!

Niyama 2 – santoṣa

This is having contentment with yourself and whatever circumstances you are in. It's about being happy and grateful for what you have and what you have been given. This is important because if we are always wanting more, then we will never be satisfied. Also, when we are constantly focused on our desires or outcomes, it's easy to lead ourselves into a state of feeling anxious.

Of course, we all have moments where it can be difficult to shift our perspective to one of appreciation, but the acceptance we cultivate through a regular practice of **santoṣa** can be life-changing, as it can help us avoid negative feelings of doubt, judgement, jealousy, etc. (When we practise **santoṣa**, we can remain calm and happy even if our surroundings may seem chaotic.) Being thankful for what you have and focusing on what's going well can help you to lead a more stress-free life.

To practise

The next time you consider buying something new, take a moment to consider if you really need it. Do you already own the same item or similar that you can be grateful for instead? Could you make do with what you have? Alternatively, are you able to truly appreciate and feel immense gratitude for everyday things like a home-cooked meal, a warm house, the clothing you own or the people in your life? Think about how these things bring you joy in your day-to-day life.

Niyama 3 – tapas

This literally translates to 'heat' or 'burn'. The practice of **tapas** includes doing things that might be challenging because, in the long run, they are good for you. Like self-discipline, **tapas** is about doing things even when you might not feel like it. When we choose things that are good for us, even when they require a lot of effort, we build inner strength and resilience.

You can see **tapas** as a practice that helps us to overcome procrastination or laziness, too. If you set yourself a goal, confront challenges or do things that are good for your mind and body it can sometimes make you feel uncomfortable, but will be better for you overall. For instance, going to the gym can prove challenging for so many of us but staying committed to your goal of going once a week can help you become fitter or healthier. It's like igniting that inner fire and using it to destroy any impurities of the mind or thoughts that might be holding you back.

Traditional types of **tapas** include:

- **Kāyika tapas** (**tapas** of the body) – The focus on building physical discipline by purifying the body, for example through fasting or altering eating habits.
- **Vāchika tapas** (**tapas** of speech) – The purification of speech through avoiding any harmful words.
- **Mānasika tapas** (**tapas** of the mind) – The practice of taming negative thought patterns through techniques like meditation.

To practise

When something proves to be challenging or you feel like giving up, see if you can persevere and show up for yourself. Visualise igniting that inner energy while keeping the ultimate purpose of your actions firmly in sight. Think of the things that give you the energy to push through difficulties and know that when you do push through it will be worth it.

Niyama 4 – svādhyāya

Svādhyāya is self-study through yogic texts and scriptures or **sādhanā** (daily spiritual practice). When **svādhyāya** is practised regularly it helps us understand our beliefs, our judgements, our emotions, our thoughts, our behaviours and our reactions better. Essentially, it helps us understand why we do the things we do.

This study of the Self in this way encourages self-reflection, personal growth and mindfulness. In addition, studying the yogic texts helps us to resonate more with the divine and to adopt teachings that can help us to evolve spiritually. **Svādhyāya** is never about judging yourself; it's about becoming a better version of yourself as yoga encourages you to do.

To practise

Make a habit of setting aside some quiet time once a week (or once a day if you can). Use this time to study yogic texts or scriptures, or reflect and write down your thoughts and feelings openly and honestly. Question your beliefs, try to understand your emotional reactions and write down what you could learn from any situation, good or bad. Gradually, you will become aware of your thoughts and behaviours, whether positive or negative, and will be able to change them if you need to.

Niyama 5 – īśvarapraṇidhānā

This is having faith in and surrendering to the divine. It's about letting go of your control over situations and outcomes, and instead trusting in whatever higher power you believe in to seize control. Like **Bhakti** yoga (see p. 123), this practice encourages us to have complete faith in that higher power so we can let go of any worries or expectations we have surrounding an outcome.

You could say that this is a practice of letting go. Letting go of attachments, ego or stress. When we release attachments to all these things, we are ultimately saying that we trust that whatever happens will happen for the best. Trusting that everything happens for a reason can be super difficult, especially during challenging times. But this principle teaches that accepting where we are and connecting to that higher power will serve a greater purpose.

Think of it as feeling held and supported throughout your journey by a higher power. Acknowledging this divine presence in your life will help you to release control and cultivate calmness.

To practise

Set aside some time to reflect on and write down anything that you might be worried about. What are your expectations of the situation? Do you feel like you need to control the outcome? Are thoughts coming up like 'What if I am not good enough?' or 'Will it work out?' or 'What if they don't like me?' Then write down the opposite of those thoughts, for example, what would happen if it did work out or how would it feel if you didn't worry about people liking you? Take a few moments to reflect. Then close your eyes for a few minutes while trying to let go.

A summary of yamas and niyamas

Both **yamas** and **niyamas** serve as tools to encourage us to live better and to develop into the best version of ourselves. However, this doesn't happen in a linear fashion, and it takes time, so patience is key.

In our effort to shift our perspectives, we can be met with challenging emotions but it's our dedication and progress that matters most. Remember, you don't have to dive in deep and try to practise all these yoga principles and practices at once. Instead, I suggest you try out the practices new to you one at a time, or only a few at a time, and repeat the same one/s over a period to see what works for you. This way, you will stop yourself from feeling overwhelmed and will be able to grasp each concept better.

Keep in mind that it's equally important to uphold these principles when no one else is looking. True change isn't effective if it's limited to public displays or aimed at impressing others. The work we do behind closed doors holds just as much significance.

A moment of introspection

The first two limbs of **Aṣṭāṅga** yoga have given us a lot of ideas to think about. Let's reflect:

- What is one practice from Limb 1 you want to try?
- What is one practice from Limb 2 you want to try?

9

Limb 3: Āsana (physical postures)

The third limb we will study is **āsana**, which allows us to reflect on the physical part of our life. We have mentioned this limb quite a bit throughout our journey already, so I'm sure a lot of you are fairly familiar with the term. But for those who need a reminder: **āsana** refers to the physical postures in yoga.

You may be wondering why this chapter on **āsana** is so long given that I've explained that physical poses make up such a small part of traditional yoga. Well, it's longer than the other sections on the eight limbs because I want to spend quite a lot of time covering the theory on **āsana** before getting into the practical exercises. This is important because although many of you will be familiar with the poses described here, it's the background context that is so often left out of modern-day teaching. Try and stay with me as much as you can because this extra information will help you get so much more out of your poses. (Plus, it's all very interesting, I promise!)

Did you know...?

There are four things that will help you enhance your **āsana** practice:

1. Patience
2. Space
3. Time
4. Acceptance

The meaning behind āsana

Āsana = 'to sit or to rest in'

Āsana has been interpreted in many different ways, but in modern yoga it's mostly seen as a series of physical postures to make us flexible. However, what most people don't know is that the purpose of these postures is actually to find stillness and comfort in a seat over a long period, so that we can eventually enter a deep meditative state. When we first try to enter a seated pose, we can often find that our legs shake, we feel pain in our ankles, our shoulders may be stiff or we experience numerous other distracting discomforts. But by practising different postures over time (i.e. different **āsanas**), we free our bodies of tension and create space within them. In turn, this space helps us to find stillness in a seated or resting position to prepare us for a deep meditative state.

You see, in yogic tradition we view the body as a vehicle for helping us to reach higher states of consciousness; nothing more. This is a valuable lesson for any beginner (or experienced practitioner!) to remember when facing **āsana**, especially if you're feeling that yoga isn't for you because you can't perform advanced physical postures. If we start looking at the postures practised during **āsana** as one element of a wider discipline, then we can hopefully begin to see **āsana** for what it is, which is much more than just a means of exercise.

Did you know...?

The number of **āsanas** taught today varies depending on the style of yoga you are practising.

For example, Sage Patañjali provides us with 12 seated meditation **āsanas** in *The Yoga Sūtras of Patañjali* (see p. 85). In contrast to this, **Haṭha** yoga tradition teaches that the **āsanas** we see today are the product of 8.4 million movements that Lord Shiva* is said to have taught to his consort Parvati, which were documented in original yogic scriptures. Yet it is then believed that while Lord Shiva taught Parvati all 8.4 million movements, Lord Shiva only taught 32 of them to everyone else. So, within **Haṭha** yoga only 32 **āsanas** are taught (although with the understanding that 8.4 million movements actually exist!).

* Lord Shiva is a Hindu deity of destruction of evil. He also symbolises inner transformation and teaches us the importance of growth and self-discipline.

The history of āsana

Yoga, in particular **āsana**, is a living tradition where generations of gurus and students have transmitted the practice orally or through the written word in India. Determining when **āsana** was first practised is tricky because dates are often lost with oral history, and many of the old sacred written texts have disappeared during past invasions. There is, though, archaeological evidence to strongly suggest that the tradition of **āsana**, or yoga postures, dates back at least 5000 years. Let me tell you now about some of the oldest known depictions of yoga that have been found in the world to date.

First, and interestingly, the earliest depictions of Lord Shiva portray him as Paśupati, the 'lord of the animals', also known as the 'horned deity'. These depictions are on statues that have been found in the Indus Valley Civilisation (a Bronze Age civilisation) at Harappa and Mohenjo-Daro (now modern-day Pakistan) (see the plate section for an image). Lord Shiva is seen here in a deep state of meditation in **Bhadrāsana** (Throne Pose). The name of this statue is the **Paśupati Seal.** The animals that are depicted around the **Paśupati Seal** are the same ones mentioned in verses of the Rig Veda (one of the oldest scriptures in Hinduism). This **Paśupati Seal** artefact gives us valuable insights into the spiritual and cultural practices of the Indus Valley Civilisation and suggests that yoga practices such as **āsana** and **dhyāna** (meditation) were a part of spiritual and religious life in ancient times.

Second, at the same site, ancient clay sculptures of figurines were found depicted engaging in various **āsanas** (along with figurines of deities and animals), which is another indicator of the presence of yoga in ancient India. Some of these artefacts may have been used for religious or decorative purposes, but today they are a key part in helping us piece together the culture of ancient India (see the plate section for an image).

The benefits of āsana

Āsana in its most traditional form, as we've discussed, provides a gateway to deep mental and spiritual transformation. However, there are many additional benefits to the practice of **āsana** today that can have a positive impact on your overall well-being: physically, mentally and emotionally, and holistically.

1. How do āsanas help us physically?

Often, **āsanas** are compared to exercises, yet the purpose of practising **āsana** differs hugely from exercise and this can be seen when we consider the two activities in relation to our *breath* and *body temperature*. While exercise typically accelerates the breath and raises body temperature, **āsana** practice encourages us to slow down our respiration, which allows our body temperature to decrease*. This intentional shift when practising **āsana** in its traditional form promotes a state of calm, which in turn helps to cultivate mindfulness and stillness. Distinguishing between these two forms of movement and their purposes plays a huge part in maintaining the integrity of yoga.

However, there are many physical benefits to practising **āsana**. For example, it:

- increases muscle strength;
- improves posture;
- aids digestion;
- detoxifies the body as it promotes circulation;
- relaxes and softens the muscles;
- reduces inflammation;
- improves balance;
- increases spinal health;
- creates healthier joints;
- improves mobility.

* Typically, during **āsana** practice, breath awareness is crucial. By consciously regulating our breath, we often bring it to a steady rhythm or slow it down. This deliberate control helps decrease oxygen levels and lowers our body temperature. There are multiple ways in which asana practice achieves this cooling effect: stimulating the parasympathetic nervous system, regulating sweat and its evaporation, promoting muscle relaxation, and enhancing blood circulation. When these elements come together in our practice, they create a noticeable cooling effect on our bodies. See *Asana Pranayama Mudra Bandha* by Swami Satyananada Saraswati (Bihar School of Yoga, 2013)

2. How do āsanas help us mentally and emotionally?

Many yogic texts explain the significance of practising **āsana** to gain control over the mind, body and nervous system, and **āsanas** are designed to target specific parts of the body and nervous system. They can therefore have a profound impact on us in terms of inducing a state of calm and helping us to regulate ourselves. Regular practice of **āsana** can:

- reduce stress;
- release tension;
- increase awareness (... of ourselves, our surroundings, of others around us etc.);
- induce mental clarity;
- improve sleep;
- reduce symptoms of anxiety and depression;
- improve focus;
- ... and many more!

The nervous system

Let's take a quick look at the nervous system and explain how we can use **āsana** and other yogic practices to support it. (Quick disclaimer: the brain is an incredibly complex system, so I'll be providing only a brief summary to help simplify the nervous system for the context of what we are addressing within yoga.)

Think of your body as a multifaceted machine with many complex wires and connections. The nervous system is like the control centre for communication that helps with the smooth running and functioning of sending and receiving messages to different parts of the body. It is a part of our body that helps to keep us balanced and safe, and it is responsible for our thoughts, actions and reactions. There are two parts to our nervous system:

1. **Central nervous system (CNS)** – This is made up of two main parts: the brain and the spinal cord. Your brain is responsible for how you think, learn and move. Your spinal cord carries messages between your brain and the rest of the body.
2. **Peripheral nervous system (PNS)** – This includes divisions called the 'somatic nervous system' and the 'autonomic →

nervous system', which are responsible for the voluntary control of skeletal muscles as well as the involuntary regulation of bodily functions, such as your heart rate, digestion and respiration.

The autonomic nervous system consists of the sympathetic and parasympathetic nervous systems. The sympathetic nervous system activates our fight-or-flight response, and the parasympathetic nervous system is linked to a rest-and-digest state. The parasympathetic nervous system contains neurons that are connected to the vagus nerve. Stimulating your vagus nerve can help you feel calm and relaxed by slowing down your heart rate. This nerve plays a crucial role in returning your body to a peaceful state when you're stressed or anxious. Yogic practices provide us with ways to stimulate the vagus nerve, which brings us back into a state of regulation.

An important aspect to remember when it comes to the nervous system and yoga is that we shouldn't be placing too much stress on our bodies in **āsana** or **prāṇāyāma** (breath control) practices. For example, forcing yourself into an **āsana** when your body isn't ready yet is more likely to activate your sympathetic nervous system and send you into fight-or-flight mode.

3. How do āsanas help us holistically?

In yoga, the mind and body aren't perceived as separate entities; they are interconnected. A primary way in which **āsanas** can help us holistically therefore is through the use of physical movements to release stagnant energy and tension within the body. These 'blockages' may be hindering us on the path to enlightenment and, when they're unblocked, they can help balance the mind and body. Untangling these knots or blockages can be seen as a way of being able to direct the flow of energy around the body, which in turn will help you to gain steadiness within your mind, body and emotions.

In yogic terms, these blockages of energy or tension in our body are called **granthis** (psychic knots), and these prevent the flow of **prāṇa** (vital energy) through our energy centres or our **chakras** (see p. 147). These **granthis** are located at different points in the Subtle Body (see p. 143) and can often cause disturbances within the mind, which can affect our daily lives. Although we cannot see these **granthis**, the impact they have can often be *felt* (especially if you're someone who is aware of certain people's auras, or even your own).

These **granthis** that form in our minds can often manifest on a physical level in the form of stress or tension in the body, and yoga offers us a toolkit to help us ease this tension and stiffness found in the mind and body. The toolkit includes a combination of **āsana**, **prāṇāyāma** and **dhyāna**, and it's interesting to note that every mental knot has a physical counterpart and vice versa. By this I mean that there is an **āsana** that exists that is specifically designed to help us address the problems of each **granthi**.

Combining **āsana**, **prāṇāyāma** and **dhyāna** helps us work on untangling these **granthis**. This then restores the balance between the mind and body and eventually leads to enhanced mental and physical strength, increased inner peace and a sense of harmonious well-being.

It's normal to feel overwhelmed when dealing with mental, physical or emotional challenges. Starting with simple practices like **āsana** or **prāṇāyāma** can be the first step towards releasing these tensions. If you need help, you can always ask a teacher. Don't be discouraged! I've outlined the concept of **granthis** to provide context and help you understand how practising **āsana** can benefit you in various aspects of your life.

Advice before you start

Before we begin talking about the specific **āsanas**, I'd like to share some general advice for anyone approaching the physical moves. This will be new information for some and a refresher for others, but it's all important to consider before beginning your **āsana** practice.

The importance of working to the level of your ability

Sometimes knowing where to begin with **āsana** can be a little daunting because of the different labels (or descriptions) that we see when looking for a class, whether it be online or in person. When approaching a class, you might see 'beginner', 'intermediate' or 'advanced' in the description, but these labels aren't always fitting. For example, you might see yourself as an intermediate student but may still need assistance with poses that are considered beginner, such as **Tadāsana** (Mountain Pose) or **Paścimottānāsana** (Seated Forward Fold). Therefore, it's important for teachers to ensure that the descriptions of their classes are clear so that people know what to expect. (Remember, language matters and making small changes creates a more accessible environment.)

These labels of 'beginner', 'intermediate' or 'advanced' shouldn't create divisions or exclude anyone; they were originally intended to be helpful guidelines. You aren't bound to remain in a single group exclusively. In fact, you may find yourself moving between them as you navigate your own mental and physical boundaries and capabilities. Your journey is uniquely yours and these descriptions are there to assist, not restrict. For instance, I have been practising for years but that doesn't mean that I can perform every advanced **āsana**. I very often place myself into 'beginner' (or sometimes 'intermediate') classes because I still find a lot of advanced poses very challenging, despite having practised for such a long time. And that's OK! It's always good to revisit the basics; I find it quite humbling. Some days are better than others and it's so important to listen to your body.

Remember the four things I said you would require for **āsana** at the beginning of this chapter? They were: patience, space, time and acceptance. Well, *acceptance* is one of the most important and, with respect to keeping your practice authentic, accepting where you are mentally and physically at any stage of your **āsana** practice, and on any given day, is essential.

Modifying āsanas

Speaking of working to your ability, it's also essential to mention that there are *always* variations to every **āsana** because **āsanas** can meet us wherever we are. Usually, we hear this concept being presented as a 'modification' to help support us in progressing through a class.

'Modifying' in the context of a yoga **āsana** class means making minor changes to the original pose to make it less extreme. Often, in modern yoga, this is interpreted as 'if you can't do this, do this', which can make you feel like you aren't practising 'real yoga'. This is far from the truth as modifications serve as a way of helping us to practise the same principles of that pose, but with extra care and caution. Sometimes you may feel like you don't want to take the modification, but it can be nice to know it's available for you. Common modifications can show up in the following ways:

- bend your knees;
- use a chair or a wall;
- use a different **āsana**;
- drop your knees;
- use a rolled blanket or bolster;
- add a block;
- ... and many more!

A note on adjustments

If you have taken part in a yoga **āsana** class before, you might have noticed teachers adjusting students. There are three types of adjustments: verbal, visual and physical. Verbal and visual adjustments involve teachers demonstrating how **āsanas** should be performed, and physical adjustments involve the teacher using their hands to guide the practitioner into a certain position.

The intention behind adjustments is to remove individuals from unsafe positions due to poor alignment or other factors that could lead to injury. As well as this, adjustments can provide encouragement to experience **āsanas** in alternative ways and to guide students into correct alignment. First and foremost, it's important to mention that adjustments shouldn't be made by teachers who don't have a deep understanding of anatomy and **āsanas**. Training in adjustments is vital for the safety of students.

Here are a few other things to bear in mind if you are making or receiving an adjustment:

- **Consent** – Always ask, or make sure you are being asked, before an adjustment takes place. It's essential to consider people's boundaries and not everyone is comfortable with physical touch.
- **Risk of injury** – Be mindful of past or present injuries or medical conditions. No one should be pushed past their limits during an adjustment.
- **Communication** – This is key if adjustments are a part of your practice. Voicing discomfort and listening to your body, or listening to the needs of your students, allows for safe and respectful adjustments.

→

I have never felt comfortable giving adjustments during my classes except for minor ones during **Śavāsana** (the final resting pose). I, and many other teachers, aren't fully trained in giving adjustments, and it's important to remember that they weren't commonly used in traditional yoga. This is because yoga, in particular **āsana**, was always viewed as more of a personal practice with an emphasis on self-awareness. Teachings were typically passed down orally with guidance from a knowledgeable teacher and classes in ancient times usually consisted of one to two people (although in most cases yoga was taught one-on-one). In any case, all of the above still applies whether you consider the use of adjustments or not.

The use of props

There are also certain props that we can use with **āsana** to help you get the most out of your practice*. They can provide support and stability while helping you with your alignment in **āsana**. Experienced practitioners also use props; they're not just aids for beginners. For example, I find it helpful to use a bolster in **Eka Pāda Rājakapotāsana** (One-legged Pigeon Pose) to help support my upper body. Here are some props that you may come across in your practice:

- **Straps/belts** – A band that assists with alignment and stretching that can help to avoid overstraining.
- **Bolsters** – A firm, cylinder-like cushion that is used for support and relaxation.
- **Chairs** – These are often used to help support those with limited mobility or other physical limitations.
- **Blocks** – A rectangular foam or cork block that is used to assist with balancing and extension.
- **Blankets** – These provide cushioning support to elevate or improve posture. They're also used to help with relaxation.
- **Mats** – These aren't essential to your practice but can be helpful in providing a non-slip surface while adding padding to the ground so that your joints feel comfortable and supported. You could also use a towel or a rug if a mat isn't accessible to you.

* Although these aren't necessary (see p. 50) and according to **aparigraha** we aim not to be tied to material possessions, there are certain props that we can use if we need a bit of extra help in our practice.

The importance of awareness during āsana

During my yoga teacher training, an emphasis was placed on the awareness of the breath in every movement during an **āsana** practice. **Aṣṭāṅga** yoga knows this as the method of **vinyāsa**, which means the synchronisation of breath with movement. Although popular modern yoga styles depict '**Vinyāsa** Yoga' as a fast-paced dynamic class, traditionally this method of **vinyāsa** encourages us to breathe deeply and mindfully rather than moving quickly through each **āsana**.

The traditional approach to **vinyāsa** involves a method called **vinyāsa krama**. **Vinyāsa** means 'to place' and **krama** means 'to arrange'. In the context of yoga **āsana**, **vinyāsa krama** is a way to practise yoga **āsana** with mindfulness and intention, emphasising the connection between breath and movement. It allows us to smoothly transition from one **āsana** to another, co-ordinating each movement with the breath. For example, you might inhale as you reach your arms up, exhale as you fold forwards, and inhale again as you lift halfway up. This technique helps practitioners move through their practice seamlessly while staying attuned to their breath. It's believed in traditional yoga that without this conscious connection to the breath during **āsana** practice, it's not truly yoga. So, **vinyāsa krama** not only keeps your body moving fluidly, but also keeps you grounded in the present moment through the rhythm of your breath.

However, remaining aware in your practice won't always be smooth sailing, especially to begin with. So, **Aṣṭāṅga** also offers the system of **tristhāna,** which we can loosely translate to 'three key places of attention'. Being guided by these three focus points helps us to concentrate and stay mindful during practice. They are:

1. **Prāṇāyāma** (breath control) – Control over the breath is the first point of attention, where inhales and exhales should remain steady and equal.
2. **Dṛṣṭi** (gaze – often styled as drishti) – A point of gaze that is used to keep the eyes from wandering during yoga practices. This helps to keep the focus directed on us rather than what's happening around us. For example, in **Adho Mukha Śvānāsana** (Downward-facing Dog), we are encouraged to place our **dṛṣṭi** at our navels. (See the following box for the nine traditional **dṛṣṭis**.)

3. **Āsana** (physical poses) - Focus on our alignment. As we pay attention to our posture, we reduce the risk of injury and get the most out of the **āsana**.

Using these three points of focus helps us to direct our attention inwards so that we experience yoga **āsana** in its entirety.

The nine traditional dṛṣṭis

To stay centred and focused on ourselves during **āsana** practice, we're guided to use nine traditional focal points for our gaze:

1. **Nāsāgra dṛṣṭi** - tip of the nose
2. **Bhrūmadhya dṛṣṭi** - between the brows where our Third Eye is
3. **Nābhi chakra dṛṣṭi** - navel
4. **Hastagram dṛṣṭi** - hands or fingertips
5. **Padayoragram dṛṣṭi** - feet or toes
6. **Ūrdhva dṛṣṭi** - upward
7. **Aṅguṣṭhamadhyam dṛṣṭi** - thumbs
8. **Pārśva dṛṣṭi** - far right or over the shoulder
9. **Pārśva dṛṣṭi** - far left or over the shoulder

Yoga attire

One of the common questions that many yoga students have is 'What should I wear for my yoga practice?' Often this is related to the practice of **āsana**, so I will include this here. What to wear is definitely a matter of personal choice, but I will let you in on what ancient yogis would wear to practise in, too.

Traditionally, yoga clothing didn't involve 'yoga pants' (that's a term coined primarily for the purposes of marketing in the Western world). In fact, Western yoga pants are really quite far removed from the inexpensive, breathable, loose cotton outfits that have been the norm in India since ancient times. Yoga practitioners there have preferred **dhotis** or **sarees** and continue to do so. This is because materials that are tight, especially around the chest or abdominal area, are more likely to restrict the breath. Losing this connection to your breath during an **āsana** practice takes away from the point of practising yoga in its entirety.

A **dhoti** is a traditional loose piece of clothing that takes the shape of your lower body while comfortably draping around your waist. **Dhotis** are comfortable and flexible and allow us to move without being restricted, which is why they are suitable for yoga practices. They also hold religious and cultural significance as they have been worn (*mostly* by men) across India for daily wear or religious ceremonies and rituals. While there is a specific way of wearing and folding the **dhoti**, which can take some getting used to, you can find modern styles that resemble the traditional garment without the complexity. A **dhoti** aligns with the yogic principles of humility and contentment, providing coverage while preserving a sense of openness and freedom. **Dhotis** are also, of course, embraced by women.

For my **āsana** practice, I personally like clothing that is well-fitted but not too tight (so my body is comfortable), as I have had experiences where clothing has distracted me during my practice. For example, a baggy T-shirt covering my face in certain postures, and therefore restricting my vision is distracting, and loose pants can cause me to stumble between poses.

When it comes to selecting clothing for your practice, here are some things to consider:

- **Material** – Try to choose soft materials made from natural fibres such as cotton or linen.
- **Breathable** – Make sure that the material can absorb sweat and that it can dry quickly.
- **Tags and labels** – Itchy labels or tags can be a huge distraction, so cut them out.
- **Moveable** – Ensuring you can move and breathe easily in your clothing is the most important thing. Especially look out for waistbands that don't clench your skin or that don't roll down, causing further distractions to your practice.

Over everything, choose an outfit for your practice that is roomy, comfortable and easy to move in, so that it doesn't cause distractions.

The practice in motion

Now let's transition to the practical aspects of **āsana**. I'll guide you through what this part of yoga entails and introduce some beginner-friendly practices for you to explore.

Typically, you will find **āsanas** are grouped into different categories. These groupings are formed on the basis of the different areas of the body that we are targeting with them, and the different effects that they have on the body.

I've found these groups to be incredibly helpful because the number of **āsanas** can be overwhelming. The groups can help us understand the different poses' uses and benefits and help guide us when we're trying to select the right sequence for our practice. They can be helpful, too, for checking if certain poses align with our pace and capabilities.

Some of these groups are:

- **Warm-up āsanas** - Gentle **āsanas** that increase blood flow and loosen the muscles to prepare and awaken the body.
- **Meditative or relaxing āsanas** - These are restorative, and usually done while seated or lying down.
- **Seated āsanas** - Carried out while sitting on the ground.
- **Standing āsanas** - Carried out while standing on your feet.
- **Supine āsanas** - Carried out while lying on your back.
- **Balancing āsanas** - These challenge your stability and balance.
- **Prone āsanas** - Carried out while lying on the front of the body.
- **Twisting āsanas** - Involves twisting the upper body.
- **Inversions** - Where the head is placed below the heart or hips in an upside-down position.

Establishing your **āsana** practice at a level that suits your body, as we discussed on p. 114, is key to ensuring that you reap the full benefits from the practice. Attempting advanced postures without a proper warm-up, for example, or without having worked on the foundational poses first, is more likely to result in injury. It could also lead to you abandoning your practice in frustration if you attempt certain poses without having mastered the basics first. So, it's always wise to make sure you ease yourself into **āsanas**, even if this simply means beginning with some poses from the gentle warm-up or meditative categories, like the ones I'm about to introduce you to. By beginning with the simplest postures, you can loosen up your muscles to make sure the body is ready to gradually progress to more difficult ones.

These categories of poses can also act as stepping stones to begin your yoga journey. They will provide you with a solid foundation for your practice, and they can be easily practised alongside the **prāṇāyāma** (breath control) practices that I will guide you through on p. 191. I have also chosen to highlight **Śavāsana** (Corpse Pose) and **Sūrya Namaskāra** (Sun Salutations), as these are two practices that I think every practitioner should know.

Warm-up āsanas

The **āsanas** in this category can help to set the foundation for your practice by warming up the muscles in your body. They can be used before a full sequence or individually by practising each one for 1 to 3 minutes.

1. Tadāsana

(ta-DAH-SAH-na) (Mountain Pose)

Stand on a flat surface and bring your feet as close together as you can, allowing your big toes and heels to touch each other. Firmly ground your feet and toes down, inhale and slightly pull your kneecaps up so that the muscles in the legs are engaged. Distribute the weight of your body evenly, not allowing it to sway to one side or the other. Draw your belly in as much as you can and push the chest slightly forwards. Stand tall and, in one line, bring your arms by the sides of your body with your palms facing forwards. Close your eyes or keep them open and breathe here for as long as you feel comfortable.

ACCESSIBLE VARIATION

Use a wall for support by standing with your back against it. Focus on your alignment and awareness of the breath. If your feet don't touch, don't worry, just keep them hip-width apart.

BENEFITS

This pose lengthens, tones and stretches the entire body. It also increases body awareness and improves focus, concentration and posture. **Tadāsana** also relaxes the nervous system and can help you to become aware of how you stand, so that you aren't leaning to one side, which can later contribute to other health conditions such as sciatica or nerve compression.

2. Prasarita Bālāsana

(pra-sa-REE-tah bah-LAHS-un-nah) (Wide-Legged Child's Pose)

Begin by sitting in a kneeling position on a flat surface like the ground or your mat. Move your knees slightly apart while keeping your bottom touching your feet. Gradually continue to move your knees until they are hip-width apart or wider. Place your big toes together and inhale as you reach your arms up. Exhale and fold forwards, extending your arms out in front as you reach the floor. Allow your abdomen to move towards your thighs or the ground or as low as your body takes you. The more you lengthen your arms, the more your chest and torso will lower down. Take deep inhales and exhales for 30 seconds or stay for up to 3 minutes.

ACCESSIBLE VARIATION

If your feet don't touch your heels, place a rolled-up blanket or a bolster between your bottom and your feet. Use a bolster or some cushions to support your torso when folding forwards if your upper body doesn't come down all the way to the floor. Alternatively, you can come down on to your elbows instead. For extra support for the neck and shoulders, place blocks under each palm or rest your forehead on a block. You can also stack the blocks and bolsters and lean forwards on to them to help your upper body reach forwards.

BENEFITS

Prasarita Bālāsana opens the hips and stretches the entire back. It deactivates your stress response and helps to balance emotions. It also stimulates the parasympathetic nervous system (see p. 169) and can help alleviate menstrual cramps.

3. Mārjāyāsana Bitilāsana

(mar-jar-YAH-sah-nah bit-ee-LAH-sah-nah) (Cat/Cow)

Bring yourself into a tabletop position on the ground. Stack your hands under your shoulders, shoulder-width apart, and your knees under the hips, hip-width apart. Keep the spine neutral to begin with and start to distribute the weight of your body evenly. Inhale and slowly begin to open your chest, drawing the belly towards the earth. As you do this your tailbone will also lift as the pelvis tilts. Lift your head and keep your **dṛṣṭi** (gaze) towards the tip of your nose. Hold for a breath and then exhale and draw the navel towards the spine as you press your hands into the ground, as if you are pushing the floor away from you. Release your head, drawing your chin towards your chest, and keep your **dṛṣṭi** towards your navel. Hold for a breath and then continue slowly working through both movements. Stay tuned with the breath and repeat for 5 to 10 rounds.

ACCESSIBLE VARIATION

Place a blanket under your knees for extra support. You can also practise in a seated position on a chair or on the ground using your forearms. This would be helpful for anyone with wrist issues or injuries, instead of using your hands.

BENEFITS

Strengthens the spine and releases tension in the upper and lower back as well as increasing the mobility of the spine. **Mārjāyāsana Bitilāsana** improves the circulation of the spinal fluid and stimulates the vagus nerve. It helps to nourish the entire nervous system.

4. Skandha Chakra

(skuhn-dhaa chuh-k-RUH (Shoulder Socket Rotation)

Sit in a comfortable seated position on a chair or on the floor. Bring your fingertips to your shoulders with your elbows facing out to each side, in line with the shoulders. Keep the spine straight as you sit upright and begin to inhale as you take your elbows all the way round in a big circle clockwise. Exhale and try to touch your elbows to your chest as they come forwards. Inhale as you rotate your elbows up and exhale as you bring them down. Repeat for 10 rounds clockwise and 10 rounds anticlockwise.

ACCESSIBLE VARIATION

If the strain is too much with your hands on your shoulders, place your hands on your head. If rotating your elbows in a large circle causes discomfort, make the circles smaller.

BENEFITS

This strengthens the shoulder joints and increases the range of motion in the shoulders. As this **āsana** helps to open the chest, it can also facilitate your **prāṇāyāma** (breath control) practice. **Skandha chakra** releases knots and tension in the neck and shoulder area and increases **prāṇa** (vital energy) throughout the body.

Meditative or relaxing āsanas

The following **āsanas** can be practised and worked on individually, without the need to carry out an entire yoga sequence. So, if you were looking to practise just a few postures to create space internally, before meditating or just to find some stillness, these can be beneficial.

1. Sukhāsana

(soo-KAH-suh-nah) (Easy Pose)

Sit on a flat surface with your legs stretched out in front of you, and then inhale and cross your legs, bending both knees. Place your right foot under your left thigh and your left foot under your right thigh. Try not to cross too tightly, so just where your feet meet your shins. Place your hands on your knees with the palms facing up or down. Relax your entire body and drop your shoulders if you find they have crept up towards your ears. Lift and lengthen through the spine as much as you can and try to keep the head, neck and spine tall and in line throughout this **āsana**. Stay here for 5 to 10 breaths while focusing on the navel area.

ACCESSIBLE VARIATION

If you find it difficult to cross your legs because they feel stiff, take your knees wider to create more space in the hips. Alternatively, place blocks or cushions under your knees or place a blanket under your sit bones. For anyone with knee pain, place rolled-up socks behind the knees. The same effect of posture can be achieved by sitting against a wall with the legs extended and then slowly bringing your feet closer to your body.

BENEFITS

Sukhāsana increases our awareness and helps us with our alignment and posture. It also relaxes the nervous system, balances emotions and calms the mind. It's a great **āsana** overall for facilitating meditation practices as it helps to keep the body alert when we are in this upright position.

When this **āsana** is practised for the first time, or even in the morning, you may experience stiffness due to lack of movement in the body. This could also be the case after extensive periods of fitness training. For example, after a long cycling session or a leg-day workout at the gym. But not to worry, there are always ways to modify!

2. Dhyāna Veerāsana

(dyaw-NUH VEER-AA-suh-nuh) (Hero's Meditation Pose)

Sit comfortably on a flat surface with your legs extended out in front of you. Place the left leg under the right, bending the knee until the left heel is touching the right side of your bottom. Then bring the right leg on top of the left leg, also bending at the knee, until the right heel touches the left side of your bottom. Try to ensure that the right knee is directly on top of the left knee if it is accessible to you. Place both hands one on top of the other on the right knee or bring your hands to your feet. Keep your upper body upright and close your eyes while focusing on your **ajña** (Third Eye) **chakra**. Stay here for 30 seconds or up to 2 minutes.

ACCESSIBLE VARIATION

If you find it difficult to sit upright, place a bolster or a blanket under your hips. For a modification on the legs – if there is a gap between your knees – place a rolled-up blanket between them. Alternatively, you can practice this **āsana** with the bottom leg extended.

BENEFITS

Dhyāna Veerāsana strengthens the pelvic area, improves digestion and stretches the outer thighs. It also increases focus and concentration during meditation.

3. Swastikāsana

(swa-uh-st-ihk-AA-suh-nuh) (Auspicious Pose)

Sit on the ground with your legs extended out in front of you and keep your upper body in an upright position. Bend your left leg at the knee until the sole of your foot touches your inner right thigh. Now bend your right leg at the knee and place your foot between your left thigh and your calf. Lengthen the spine and place your hands on your knees, then stay here for 1 to 3 minutes while taking deep inhales and exhales. If it feels comfortable, you can stay in the pose for up to 10 minutes.

ACCESSIBLE VARIATION

If it is difficult to place your right foot between your left thigh and calf, place your right foot in front of your left leg, resting the sole of your foot against the left shin. As a beginner, this may be challenging if you have tight hips. If this is the case, elevate your hips by sitting on a blanket. You can also place cushions underneath your knees and lean your back against a wall. If your knees aren't quite reaching the floor comfortably, that's perfectly OK. Allow them to find their natural position. The key is to honour your body's needs as you work towards greater flexibility.

BENEFITS

Swastikāsana helps to improve concentration and is a preparatory practice for **prāṇāyāma** and **dhyāna** (meditation). It also calms and soothes the nervous system and can aid with digestion as it restricts blood flow in the lower limbs. By reducing inflammation in the veins and legs, this **āsana** is also said to reduce varicose veins. While in this **āsana**, the **nāḍīs** (energy channels) at the back of the legs are also stimulated.

4. Vajrāsana

(va-jr-AA-suh-nuh) (Thunderbolt Pose)

This **āsana** can be used as an alternative to the previous pose, **Swastikasana** (Auspicious Pose). **Vajrāsana** is practised by kneeling on the floor with your knees as close together as possible. Allow your big toes to touch while leaving space between both heels. Your heels will touch the sides of your hips as you sit in the gap between the heels and ankles. Keep your upper body in an upright position and allow your hands to rest on your lap with the palms facing down. Focus on your breath, deeply inhaling and exhaling. Stay here for 10 breaths or as long as you feel comfortable.

ACCESSIBLE VARIATION

If you feel discomfort in your knees or ankles while seated in this position, place a rolled-up blanket under your ankles and knees and a block between your feet. If discomfort is felt in your knees, a cushion or a bolster can also be placed under your hips. Alternatively, a rolled-up blanket between the back of the knees can take pressure off them, too.

BENEFITS

This **āsana** helps in distributing the flow of **prāṇa** through our **nāḍīs** so that we can internally heal the body. The purpose of keeping the knees together is to help keep the thighs firm and supported rather than dropping them between the feet, which also helps the flow of **prāṇa**. **Vajrāsana** improves circulation around the body and is said to be the best **āsana** to practise while meditating for those who suffer from sciatica.

Although it's generally recommended that **āsana** should be practised on an empty stomach, it's advised to practise **Vajrāsana** after meals as it is believed to improve digestion, and the pressure of the big toes touching activates the **nāḍīs**, which in turn improves digestion.

Śavāsana

(sh-uv-AA-suh-nuh)

The most important of all the **āsanas** is another meditative or relaxing posture called **Śavāsana**. The ancient yogic text *Gheranda Samhita* by

Swami Niranjananda Saraswati refers to **Śavāsana** as '**Mritasana**' which translates to 'Death Pose'. This is to signify the death of the ego or to diminish the sense of 'I am the body', and this is essentially what we are trying to achieve through the practice of **Śavāsana**.

Śavāsana is typically practised at the end of a yoga session. This is because after moving our bodies in **āsana** or practising **prāṇāyāma** we need rest to help regulate our nervous system. This part of the practice is skipped by many people, either because they find it uncomfortable to find stillness here or simply because they are finished with the physical practice and don't feel this part is relevant.

I'd like to clarify that practising **Śavāsana** is essential to your practice. It is very much more than just an **āsana**; it is a practice in itself. It helps us to rest our minds and bodies, to develop awareness of the body and to reduce fatigue. It is said that missing out on this practice can cause our minds to become agitated throughout the day, especially after a strenuous practice. If you normally experience discomfort in **Śavāsana**, I invite you to follow the instructions below now (with your eyes open or your gaze softened) and see if you are able to find some comfort this time.

Practising Śavāsana

Although **Śavāsana** is usually practised at the end of a yoga class, you can practise it any time you feel like you need a bit of rest and recovery. It can, in fact, be just as effective if practised between dynamic practices or even just before you go to sleep at night. Simply follow the steps below:

1. Lie flat on your back with your legs out straight and your arms relaxed by your sides, slightly away from your body. An option is to place a rolled-up blanket or a bolster underneath your knees here. (I also like to place a blanket over me and cover my eyes with an eye pillow.)
2. Relax your shoulders and lift your head up as you draw your chin towards your chest before placing it back down.
3. Close your eyes and listen to the natural rhythm of your breath.
4. Allow your body to feel heavy and grounded.
5. Stay connected to the breath, paying particular attention to your exhales. Every time you exhale, see this as an opportunity to relax every muscle in your body.

6. Notice any sensations that might be coming up for you.
7. Allow your body to be exactly as it is and stay in this position for 5 to 7 minutes.
8. Before opening your eyes or moving, notice how you are feeling.
9. Awaken your body by moving your fingers and toes, circle your ankles and wrists, and move your head from side to side.
10. Take a stretch with your arms above your head and roll on to your right side, curling up into a foetal position before slowly bringing yourself back up to a seated position.

Tips on practising Śavāsana

Emphasis is placed on the correct position during this practice, to avoid falling asleep. If you are simply lying down, it's likely that you won't benefit from the practice entirely. The yogic text *Gheranda Samhita* explains that the ideal placement of the hands and feet is as follows:

> 'The distance between the feet should be equal to the width of the waist. If the waist is 30 cm wide, the distance between the feet should also be 30 cm wide. The arms should be about 15 cm away from the body. The palms should be open and facing upward, allowing the fingers to curl slightly.'
>
> – *Gheranda Samhita* by Swami Niranjananda Saraswati

Swami Niranjananda Saraswati then goes on to explain that movement should be avoided in this position, to maintain awareness of the body and to avoid the desire to fall asleep. Focus should be kept on the breath or by bringing awareness to each part of the body, as we do during a **Yoga Nidrā** practice (see p. 211).

Benefits

When practised mindfully, we can benefit from **Śavāsana** in many ways. In short, **Śavāsana** is like a reset button for your nervous system as it allows your body to rest and digest. It is effective at: reducing stress and tension in the mind and body; helping us to relax; enhancing mental clarity; and encouraging deep relaxation, which can help to calm the sympathetic nervous system and activate the parasympathetic nervous system (see p. 169).

A note on inversions

Although handstands and headstands are the most common inversions that we see (especially when it comes to social media), inversions in yoga are in fact *any posture where the head is placed below the heart or hips in an upside-down position.* In short, any posture where your heart is higher than your head is considered an inversion in yoga. Often, people shy away from inversions as they think of them as intense balancing postures that require great strength, but that's simply not the case.

I am here to tell you that being able to carry out an inversion doesn't have to involve balancing on your hands or head. I won't be going into detail with inversions here (as I'd like you to focus on the 'warm-up **āsana**' and 'meditative or relaxing **āsana**' groups first), but I wanted to mention them so you can try them out when you're ready.

There are a variety of inversions that beginners can practise that have the same effect as headstands and handstands, but without the difficulty factor. Here are some beginner-friendly inversions that you can try out (you may already even practise some of them):

- **Viparītakaraṇī** - Legs Up the Wall
- **Adho Mukha Śvānāsana** - Downward-facing Dog
- **Ardha Pincha Mayurāsana** - Dolphin Pose
- **Pādāṅguṣṭhāsana** - Hand to Big Toe Pose

Sūrya Namaskāra

(soo-REE-yuh nam-uh-SKAA-ruh) (Sun Salutations)

Sūrya Namaskāra is a sequence of **āsanas**, commonly called Sun Salutations, which help awaken the mind and body. The rhythmic sequence consists of 12 **āsanas** and each breath is linked with a movement (see p. 191 for more on **prāṇayama**). The practice of **Sūrya Namaskāra** is not limited to one style of yoga or philosophy; it has such a rich history.

Sūrya Namaskāra is now practised as a tool to build strength, flexibility and balance within the mind and body. Originally, though, during the Vedic period, the purpose of this practice was to welcome a new day via the sun, which symbolises God. **Sūrya** means 'sun' and **namaskāra** means 'greeting', which in this context means to 'greet the sun'. During this time **Sūrya Namaskāra** was not carried out in the form of movement (as it is today) but through **mantras** that were chanted by a priest.

How to practise Sūrya Namaskāra*

As a beginner, you may find practising **Sūrya Namaskāra** helpful as a warm-up to your **āsana** practice, or as a way of beginning your day while focusing on cultivating gratitude. It can be practised at any time of the day, although it's believed that the period around sunrise is the best time to revitalise the body. Whenever you choose to do it, simply follow the steps below:

1. **Prānamāsana** (Prayer Pose) – Stand up straight with your feet as close together as possible, balancing your weight equally on both feet. Relax your shoulders. Inhale and bring the palms of your hands together in front of your chest as you exhale.
2. **Hasta Uttānāsana** (Raised Arms Pose) – Inhale, lifting your arms towards the sky, slightly arching your back.
3. **Hastapādāsana** (Hand to Foot Pose) – Exhale, bending forwards to touch the floor or your shins. If your hands don't touch the floor with your legs straight, take a slight bend at the knees.
4. **Ashwa Sanchalanāsana** (Equestrian Pose) – Inhale, stepping your right leg back into a lunge position.
5. **Daṇḍāsana** (Plank Pose) – Inhale, stepping your left leg back to a plank position.
6. **Aṣṭāṅga Namaskāra** (Eight-limbed Pose) – Exhale, lowering your knees, chest and forehead to the floor.
7. **Bhujaṅgāsana** (Cobra Pose) – Inhale, lifting your chest while keeping your hands and feet on the ground.
8. **Adho Mukha Śvānāsana** (Downward-facing Dog) – Exhale, lifting your hips towards the sky, forming an inverted V shape.

* If you have practiced **Sūrya Namaskāra** before, it's worth noting that the practice described here is the classical **Haṭha** version. You might be familiar with the more modern Aṣṭāṅga Vinyasa version, which has a few differences in the **āsanas**.

9. **Ashwa Sanchalanāsana** (Equestrian Pose) – Inhale, stepping your right foot between your hands into a lunge.
10. **Hastapadāsana** (Hand to Foot Pose) – Exhale, bringing your left foot forwards to meet the right, and bring your hands to the floor.
11. **Hasta Uttānāsana** (Raised Arms Pose) – Inhale and take your arms up, bringing them into a prayer position. Take a slight backbend.
12. **Tadāsana** (Mountain Pose) – Exhale and straighten your body while bringing your arms by your sides.

This completes half a round of **Sūrya Namaskāra**. Repeat on the left side by stepping your left foot back first to complete a full round. Practise 5 to 10 times.

Benefits

Practising **Sūrya Namaskāra** can have the following benefits:

- stimulates the nervous system;
- helps with blood circulation;
- increases strength and flexibility;
- strengthens muscles and joints;
- boosts your immune system.

Book resources for āsana

Desikachar, T. K. V., *The Heart of Yoga* (Inner Traditions, 1995)
Mohan, A. G., *Yoga for the Body, Breath, and Mind* (Shambhala Publications Inc, 1993)
Saraswati, Swami Niranjananda, *Gheranda Samhita* (Bihar School of Yoga, 2012)
Muktibodhananda, Swami, *Haṭha Yoga Pradīpikā* (Bihar School of Yoga, India, 1998)

A moment of introspection

This has probably been a lot to take in! But it's valuable to understand how we can integrate **āsana** into our broader yoga practice. I suggest you take some time now to digest the new information and reflect on what you've read by considering the following:

- What did you learn about **āsana** that was unfamiliar to you before? Write down any newfound insights.
- If you previously viewed yoga as a primarily physical practice, have you experienced any shift in perspective from reading this part of the book? If so, how so?
- What's one next step you can take to integrate something you've learned here into your current practice?

10

Limb 4: Prāṇāyāma (regulation of breath)

Understanding prāṇāyāma

Before we begin, take a deep breath in through the nose for four counts, 1 ... 2 ... 3 ... 4. Then slowly exhale through the nose ... 4 ... 3 ... 2 ... 1.

How do you feel? I expect you may feel slightly more relaxed than before. Often, that one breath alone is enough to show you how effective **prāṇāyāma** is for our health.

In the Western world, **prāṇāyāma** is often known as 'breathwork' or 'breathing exercises'. These practices involve consciously working with the breath to reduce stress, increase relaxation and foster personal growth. While Western breathwork draws from **prāṇāyāma**, it's important to understand **prāṇāyāma** in its traditional context, too, which is what we'll be looking at here.

In yogic tradition, **prāṇāyāma** serves as the link between **āsana** (physical postures) and **dhyāna** (meditation) to guide us deeper into our practice. This is because, from a yogic and philosophical perspective, once we learn how to control our breath, we gain the ability to still the mind and become more focused in meditation. Or, as yoga teacher A. G. Mohan sums it up:

> 'When you practice it [prāṇāyāma], you deliberately change your normal pattern of breathing which, in turn, changes your state of mind. This reduces mental disturbance and minimizes the impurities in your system.'
>
> – *Yoga for the Body, Breath, and Mind* by A. G. Mohan

Traditionally, gurus wouldn't advise their students do any meditation practices (Limb 7) until they saw that they could cultivate stillness through **āsana** practices *and* regulate their breath through **prāṇāyāma**. Therefore, **prāṇāyāma** is key when it comes to our meditative practices. **Prāṇāyāma** also specifically focuses on *controlling the breath to refine our respiratory system*, which in turn nurtures our physical, spiritual, mental and emotional well-being, too.

The meaning of prāṇa

Let's look at the meaning behind the term **prāṇāyāma**. **Prāṇa** signifies 'life force' or 'vital energy' and **āyāma** means 'to regulate' or 'to extend'. So, in this context, **prāṇāyāma** means 'to regulate or extend our vital energy'. Entire books have been written on **prāṇa** but to help you grasp it more easily, let's simplify the meaning here.

Prāṇa is often referred to as 'vital energy' because the tradition of yoga teaches that energy forms the very essence of life. When we breathe, we're not just taking in air; we're also taking in **prāṇa**, which sustains us. This vital energy is what keeps us alive and vibrant. Imagine **prāṇa** as the life force that flows through us, connecting our body and consciousness. Just as a bridge connects two sides, **prāṇa** links our physical being with our inner awareness. The breath serves as the pathway for **prāṇa**, so by mastering our breath, we're also mastering our vital energy. This understanding helps us realise the profound connection between our breath, energy and overall well-being.

Prāṇāyāma practices are like gentle guides that help us tap into the natural flow of our **prāṇa**. This energy flows through our energetic body, known as **prāṇamaya koṣa** (see p. 143), bringing a sense of calmness to our mind, body and nervous system. Think of it as creating a peaceful sanctuary within ourselves, setting the stage for deeper meditation practices later on.

Understanding how to consciously direct the flow of **prāṇa** through the teachings of **prāṇāyāma** also holds the potential to influence our entire being in profound ways. These practices serve as powerful tools for clearing away any unconscious blockages that might be holding us back. Whether it's **granthis** (psychic knots, see p. 169) or **saṃskāra** (deep-seated impressions, see p. 80), **prāṇāyāma** helps us dissolve these barriers, paving the way for positive changes and behaviours. What's more, by increasing oxygen and blood circulation throughout the body, **prāṇāyāma** gives us a natural energy boost, leaving us feeling revitalised and ready for whatever comes our way.

In simple terms, **prāṇa** isn't just some abstract concept – it's present in everything we do. It's in the way we move our bodies and even in the thoughts we think. Swami Sivananda articulates this in his book *The Science of Pranayama* where he writes: 'Prana becomes visible on the physical plane as motion and action, and on the mental plane as thought.'

The practice of **prāṇāyāma**, therefore, has many benefits, including: helping us to remove unconscious blockages (at mental, physical, emotional and spiritual levels in the body); increasing our focus and concentration to prepare us for deep states of meditation; regulating our nervous system; and removing impurities, such as waste products, from the respiratory system, which can contribute to mental and physical health issues.

The four parts of breathing

In **prāṇāyāma**, there are four components of the breath that are consciously controlled to help us regulate the flow of **prāṇa** in the body. These are:

1. **Pūraka** – inhalation
2. **Rechaka** – exhalation
3. **Antar kumbhaka** – internal breath retention
4. **Bahir kumbhaka** – external breath retention

Although the four components have been categorised in this way, they are all linked, as one action cannot be performed without the others.

In yogic philosophy, it is said that the most important part of **prāṇāyāma** is **kumbhaka** (retention of the breath, i.e. numbers 3 and 4 in the list above). According to **Haṭha** yoga, there can be no **prāṇāyāma** without **kumbhaka**.

Physically, the practice of **kumbhaka** is said to increase carbon dioxide in the body, which helps us to utilise the oxygen in our bodies over time. When we practise retaining the breath, we can also retain **prāṇa** in the body and strengthen the respiratory muscles and the diaphragm. On a mental level, **kumbhaka** helps us build concentration and self-awareness. It activates the parasympathetic nervous system (see p. 169), eventually reducing stress levels. However, it's important to mention that **kumbhaka** is considered quite advanced and may take some time to build up to.

Before we get there, we first need to look at the two foundational practices: **pūraka** (inhalation) and **rechaka** (exhalation). Both of these play a pivotal role in altering our breath patterns (and are far safer to practise on your own); these are what the exercises at the end of this chapter will focus on. A **pūraka** during **prāṇāyāma** has a more energising effect on the mind and body as it encourages us to expand and lengthen through the chest and spine, which can help elevate our mood. However, a greater emphasis is often placed on **rechaka** during **prāṇāyāma**, as this process helps us to eliminate impurities and tension. If you were to sigh now, you would feel a sense of relief. This explains why, when we exhale, we feel calmer and more grounded.

Prāṇāyāma and mental health

Often, we hear about how **prāṇāyāma** practices can help to reduce the symptoms of stress-induced psychological disorders such as **anxiety**, **depression** and **panic attacks**. The simple act of inhaling and exhaling can have a great impact on our nervous system once we are aware of the many ways to manipulate the breath using **prāṇāyāma**.

I recently had to undergo an MRI scan for my lower back injury and the thought of being in a confined space triggered my claustrophobia. Despite my efforts to prepare in the days leading up to the scan (by intensifying my self-care routine and practising yogic breathing techniques), I couldn't prevent the panic when I entered the room. As I was positioned on the bed, the technicians began the process by slowly moving the surface I was lying on into the tunnel. I felt an immediate surge of panic and my body tensed up. My mouth became dry and I had to ask them to stop.

They did stop and came over to help me regain a calm state. It took several attempts before I felt comfortable enough to allow them to proceed again. By the time the scan was complete, I was still in a dysregulated state. However, throughout the procedure the one thing that kept me there was my understanding of the strong connection between our breath and our stress response. I consciously tapped into my breath using **prāṇāyāma** exercises, which proved valuable in helping me to endure the daunting scan. **Prāṇāyāma** provides us with tools to connect with our nervous system, enabling us to regulate it in stressful situations like the one I faced during the MRI.

How āsana supports prāṇāyāma

Yogic tradition highlights the importance of using the diaphragm as we breathe to ensure we are maximising the absorption of **prāṇa** into the lower regions of the lungs. By increasing our lung capacity through **prāṇāyāma**, we allow oxygen to circulate more freely in our bloodstream, ultimately contributing to the reduction of stress and anxiety. This explains why many yoga practices encourage abdominal breathing over breathing into the chest (as most of us naturally do). When we direct the flow of breath to the abdomen region, it's easier to engage the diaphragm effectively.

However, if we haven't been exposed to proper breath techniques, have poor posture or hold a lot of tension in our minds and bodies, conscious abdominal breathing can decrease our lung capacity. This is where our **āsana** practice can prove useful, because certain **āsanas** focus on creating space in the chest and ribcage that can complement our **prāṇāyāma** practice and help us connect to the diaphragm during breathing. This ensures we use the full capacity of our lungs. Here are a few recommended **āsanas** that can help expand your chest and ribcage, making your **prāṇāyāma** practice more effective:

- **Supported Matsyāsana** (Fish Pose)
- **Bhujaṅgāsana** (Cobra Pose)
- **Paśchimottānāsana** (Seated Forward Fold)

In short, the diaphragm plays a central role in our breathing process. As we inhale, the diaphragm moves downwards, expanding the lower lungs, and the belly gently expands. As we exhale, the diaphragm moves upwards, and the belly draws in towards the spine. These two synchronised actions enable us to take in more oxygen during the inhale and expel waste gases during the exhale. As we consciously work on this aspect of **prāṇāyāma**, we not only become more aware of our current state but we also cultivate mindfulness in our mind-body connection.

Practising prāṇāyāma

So, here are two practices that will help you to work on **pūraka** and **rechaka**, which you can also use if you ever find yourself in stressful situations like the one I shared earlier.

Usually, it's advised that the practice of **prāṇāyāma** is carried out in the early morning because that's when our body's natural energies are at their peak. By starting your day with **prāṇāyāma** you can set a strong foundation for mental, physical and spiritual well-being, helping you feel more grounded throughout the day. However, for it to fit into our modern lives, it can be practised at any time of the day as long as it's not directly after a meal (to ensure you feel comfortable and to allow for proper digestion).

To practise **prāṇāyāma**, emphasis is placed on sitting in a comfortable upright position with little to no movement. If the floor is uncomfortable, a chair is recommended. (The 'General Guidelines' listed in *Yoga for Body, Breath and Mind* by A. G. Mohan are a great starting point for beginners approaching the practice if you'd like to look into this further.)

Practice 1 – Bhramari Prāṇāyāma

(Humming Bee Breath, focusing on **pūraka** and **rechaka**)

This **prāṇāyāma** specifically activates the vagus nerve (see p. 169), which can help to reduce the chronic stress that is experienced during a panic attack. Using it will allow you to regain control over your breath, body and mind. It has been proven to reduce stress while activating the parasympathetic nervous system, facilitating a quicker recovery after stressful situations, and stimulating our rest-and-digest state.

Here's how to practise:

1. Sit yourself in a comfortable meditative **āsana** and close your eyes or soften the gaze.
2. Relax your body and ensure your lips are sealed with your teeth slightly separated.
3. Raise your arms sideways and bend your elbows, bringing your index or middle finger on the tragus (the flaps) of your ears to close them off.
4. Trying to keep your body still, inhale fully, bringing focus to the **ajña** (Third Eye) **chakra** and then exhale while making a slow, deep humming sound.

Duration: 5–10 rounds or for 2–5 minutes
Frequency: Daily

Benefits: Relieves stress and tension, increases the healing capacity of the body and has a soothing effect on the mind
Do not practice: If you have sinus problems or high blood pressure as it can increase blood pressure and pressure in the ear canal

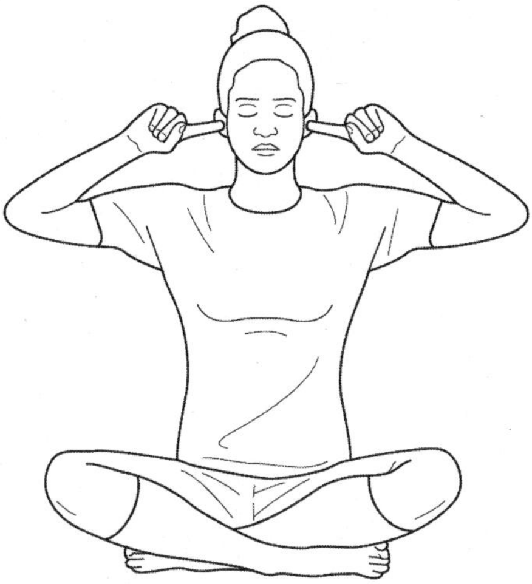

Practice 2 – Nāḍī Śodhana

(Alternate Nostril Breathing, focusing on **pūraka** and **rechaka**)

This practice is centred around purifying the energy channels as we use new **prāṇa** to balance **iḍā nāḍī** (our left energy channel) and **pingalā nāḍī** (our right energy channel) (see p. 143). **Nāḍī Śodhana** helps to soothe and regulate the autonomic nervous system and lowers stress and anxiety levels through the balance of the sympathetic and parasympathetic nervous systems (see p. 168). It can also aid in lowering blood pressure and boosting the immune system.

Here's how to practise:

1. Sit in a comfortable seated position with a straight spine. Relax your shoulders and your entire body and take a few clearing breaths.
2. Allow your left hand to rest on your left knee and bring your right hand to your nose.
3. Create **Vishnu Mudra** by drawing your index and middle finger in towards your palm and resting your ring and little finger on your left nostril. Your thumb will be used to close your right nostril.

4. Press gently on your right nostril to close it, and exhale slowly and completely through your left nostril. Then breathe in through the same nostril (left).
5. Close your left nostril with your ring and little finger and open your right nostril as you exhale slowly. Breathe in from your right nostril and then exhale from your left. This is one round of **Nāḍī Śodhana**.

Duration: 5–10 rounds or for 3–5 minutes
Frequency: Once or twice daily
Benefits: Improves focus, balances the mind and body, calms the nervous system and reduces stress and anxiety

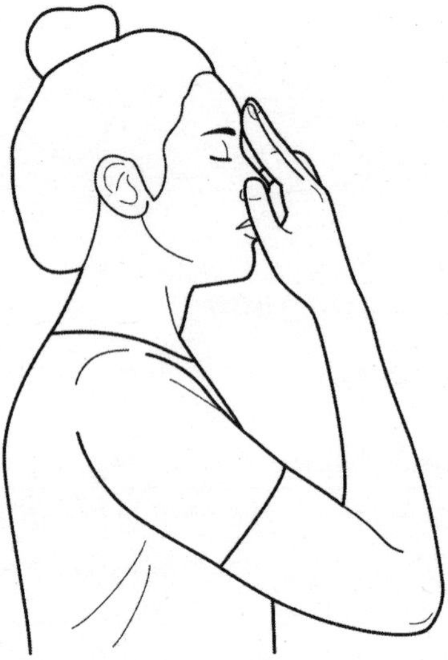

TIP

Counting your inhales and exhales equally during **prāṇāyāma** practices is helpful in terms of staying mindful of the breath. Here's how you can incorporate equal breathing into both of the practices above:

1. Try inhaling for the count of three and then exhaling for three.
2. Slowly increase the number when the practice can be carried out with ease.
3. Gradually, you will be able to increase your lung capacity and later incorporate **kumbhaka** into both methods.

Summarising prāṇāyāma

In yoga tradition, **prāṇāyāma** serves as a bridge between **āsana** and **dhyāna**, guiding us deeper into our practice. **Prāṇāyāma** works on refining our respiratory system, benefitting our physical, spiritual, mental and emotional well-being. Think of it as regulating our **prāṇa**, which sustains life itself. By consciously directing our breath, we tap into this energy flow, creating a sense of calmness and balance in our body and mind.

Learning **prāṇāyāma** takes time and patience, but its benefits are great as it can support us in stressful situations and daily life.

Book resources for prāṇāyāma

Desikachar, T. K. V., *The Heart of Yoga* (Inner Traditions, 1995)

Sivananda, Swami, *The Science of Pranayama* (Divine Life Society, 2009)

Saraswati, Swami Niranjananda, *Gheranda Samhita* (Bihar School of Yoga, 2012)

Mohan, A. G., *Yoga for the Body, Breath, and Mind* (Shambhala Publications Inc, 1993)

11

Limb 5: Pratyāhāra (the influence of our senses)

As we move through the stages of **Aṣṭāṅga**, we're essentially constructing a connection from **prakṛti** (the outside world) to **puruṣa** (our inner Self). The initial four limbs of **Aṣṭāṅga**, as a reminder, have involved external practices where we work on the physical aspects of life, while the last four limbs guide us inwards as we gradually detach from the external world.

Pratyāhāra serves as the starting point for this bridge, as this fifth limb of yoga helps us explore the 'mental' aspect of our life. It involves concentrating on a single point to help us withdraw from our senses. This limb is crucial preparation for meditation, especially for beginners or for those who find it challenging to cultivate stillness. Usually, we rely on our senses for stimulation, but this practice encourages us to do the opposite. It teaches us to disengage our minds from our senses to allow us to become fully absorbed in the present moment. By focusing our minds on one situation or object, our senses come under our control (whereas when we allow our minds to be led by our senses, our senses control us).

Let me explain how this works. Imagine that you are sitting in a peaceful park on a sunny day, feeling the warmth of the sun on your skin. Initially, your attention might be drawn towards the sound of chirping birds or the chatter of people around you. However, when you begin to focus on the sound of your breath (if this is the chosen point of focus, for example), then you gradually become more centred and present. At this point, **pratyāhāra** helps you detach from the senses that typically consume your attention, allowing you to find comfort in the simplicity of your breath.

As T. K. V Desikachar says in his book *The Heart of Yoga*, 'Precisely because the mind is so focused, the senses follow it; it is not happening the other way around.' So, by improving our ability to concentrate on a single point (in the example above it was our breathing), we reclaim control over our senses and empower ourselves to experience deep states of inner peace and awareness.

This practice aims to detach us from our sensory organs. But learning to control our senses doesn't mean we stop using them altogether as, of course, they are essential for navigating the external world. Instead, it's about knowing how and when to avoid letting our senses distract us when we need to maintain focus. As we begin to incorporate **pratyāhāra** into our lives, we begin to develop the skill of redirecting our attention inwards, away from our senses.

Sage Patañjali defines **pratyāhāra** in yoga **sūtra** 2:54, as follows:

स्वविषयासंप्रयोगे चित्तस्य स्वरूपानुकार इवेन्द्रियाणां प्रत्याहारः

svaviṣaya-asaṁprayoge cittasya svarūpānukāra-iv-endriyāṇāṁ pratyāhāraḥ

> 'The drawing in of the organs is by their giving up their own objects and taking the form of the mind-stuff.'
> – *The Yoga Sūtras of Patañjali* (2:54) by Swami Vivekananda

Here, Patañjali is suggesting that when we focus our mind inwards during meditation, our sensory organs withdraw from their usual external activities. Instead, they align with the mental state, becoming still and calm.

Learning to withdraw from our senses can also be seen as a way of learning to refrain from pursuing material objects. If we apply the dualism of **puruṣa** and **prakṛti** here, we can make more sense of it. During the state of **pratyāhāra**, we begin to realise our **puruṣa** and gain a greater insight into the unchanging aspect of it. We gradually begin to focus more inwards on self-reflection and self-awareness, and so we slowly detach our focus from the **prakṛti** and all the material possessions that come with it.

Practice – Shanmukhi Mudra

To help you become acquainted with **pratyāhāra**, here's a practice to try. **Shanmukhi Mudra** guides you through detaching from your senses so that the flow of energy goes inwards, and we can develop inner focus. This inner focus helps prepare us for meditation.

Here's how to practise:

1. Sit in a comfortable seated position, relax the body and bring awareness to your breath.
2. Close your eyes and take a few breaths.
3. Bring your palms to your face, bending the elbows so that they come out to the sides.
4. Close the flaps (the tragus) of your ears with your thumbs, place your index fingers on top of your eyes, use your middle fingers to slightly cover your nostrils, and place your ring finger tip on your upper lip and your little finger tip on your lower lip.
5. Inhale through your nose fully and then close your nostrils with your middle fingers. Listen for any sounds or vibrations within.
6. Briefly hold and then, releasing your middle fingers, slowly exhale.
7. Repeat as many times as you can, each time connecting more with the inner vibrations and staying focused on the breath.

Duration: 5–10 minutes
Frequency: Once or twice a week
Benefits: Relaxes the nervous system, soothes the muscles of the face and enhances focus and concentration

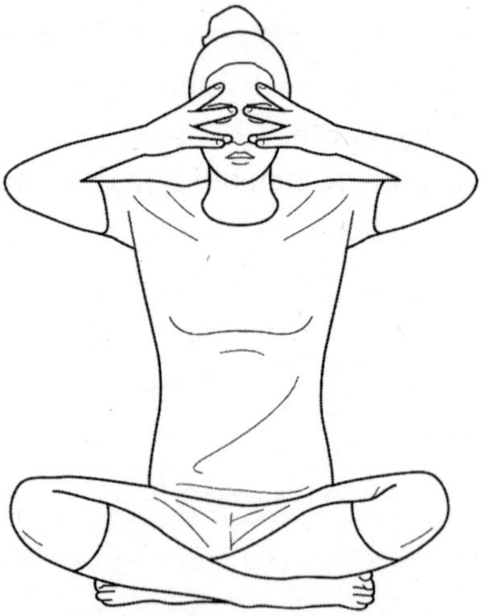

12

Limb 6: Dhāraṇā (concentration)

The previous limb, **pratyāhāra** (the influence of our senses), forms the foundation for this sixth limb of yoga, **dhāraṇā** in which we concentrate our mind or attention on a single object or meditation of our choice. This allows us to explore the psychological aspect of life.

Our aim is to immerse ourselves fully in our focal point, whether it's a single object, idea or even our breath. By anchoring our focus in this way, on one item, we create stability in the mind, which prevents it from wandering aimlessly. Although external distractions may occasionally pull our attention away, we can train ourselves to gently return to our chosen focal point.

'**Dhāraṇā** (concentration) is when the mind holds on to some object, either in the body, or outside the body, and keeps itself in that state.' – *The Yoga Sūtras of Patañjali* (3:1) by Swaṃi Vivekananda

If you notice your thoughts or emotions distracting you during meditation, then having a focal point, such as the breath, can bring you back to the present moment. As we sustain our focus on a single object, everything else around us gradually fades into the background. Of course, your mind will drift, it's only natural, but as long as we keep coming back to the chosen object, our ability to focus will enhance and awareness of the Self can be cultivated.

A note on the difference between pratyāhāra (Limb 5) and dhāraṇā (Limb 6)

To keep things clear, let's understand the difference between **pratyāhāra** and **dhāraṇā**. Both help us to prepare for meditation, but in slightly different ways. Think of **pratyāhāra** as withdrawing

→

from external distractions, a bit like turning the volume down in a busy environment. **Dhāraṇā** guides us to concentrate on one thing, similar to focusing your gaze on a single point, like zooming in on an object and fixing your attention to it.

In short, becoming completely immersed in an object of your choosing without letting outside distractions come in is how **dhāraṇā** shows up in our yoga practice.

Here are some traditional objects you could choose to focus on during this practice, but feel free to select anything that resonates with you:

- **Yantras**
- The Moon
- Flowers
- Symbols such as **om**
- Your breath
- Deities

Practice: Trāṭaka

(Candle Gazing)

Trāṭaka is where we focus all our attention on the flame of a candle to enhance our ability to focus. This practice appears in several yogic texts and is good preparation for meditation.

In the *Haṭha Yoga Pradīpikā* (see p. 86), Swami Swatmarama shares this practice with us and says: 'the impression of the flame remains for some time.' When we stare at a flame for long enough and then close our eyes, we are still able to visualise the flame.

Here's how to practise:

1. Light a candle (safely) in a dark room and place it on a flat surface at eye level. Ensure the flame remains steady and doesn't flicker too much.

2. Sit in a comfortable seat, relax the body and close your eyes as you take a few deep breaths.
3. Open your eyes and then steadily begin to gaze at the flame just above the wick. Try your best not to blink or move your eyes.
4. If you find your mind wandering, simply bring your awareness back to the practice.
5. Stare at the flame for as long as you can until you can no longer maintain your gaze.
6. Close your eyes and focus on the vision of the flame that remains once you have done this.
7. As soon as the image begins to fade, try to re-envision it until you no longer can.
8. Open your eyes and then repeat the practice if you feel comfortable.
9. Once you have completed the practice, gently place your palms on top of your eyes for a moment and then relax.

Duration: 1–2 minutes
Frequency: 2–3 rounds once a week or once every other week
Benefits: Increases focus and concentration, balances the nervous system and improves memory and vision

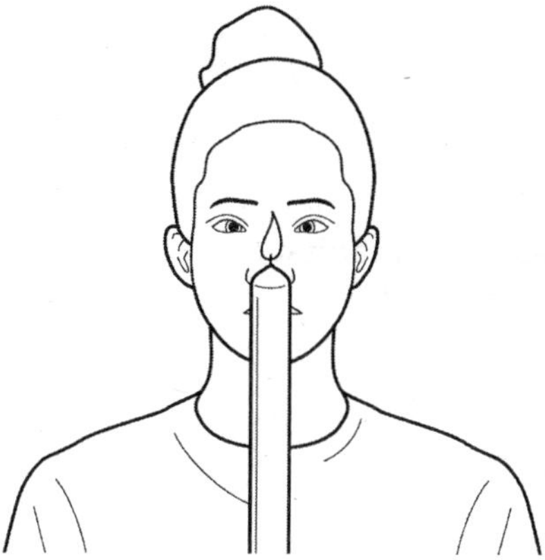

13

Limb 7: Dhyāna (meditation)

Although we can label the six previous limbs of yoga as practices, the seventh limb – **dhyāna** – isn't classified as a practice according to yogic philosophy. Instead, **dhyāna** is a *state* that is cultivated. Yoga emphasises the importance of building on the previous six limbs to ultimately lead us to cultivate a state of **dhyāna** at this point. This seventh limb allows us to explore the intellectual aspect of life.

Control of the mind is essential for spiritual evolution on the path of yoga. Sometimes we can be our own worst enemies by chasing after things that are external or out of our control. And when we fill our mind with external factors, our awareness of the Self becomes distorted. That is why meditation is so key.

बन्धुरात्मात्मनस्तस्य येनात्मैवात्मना जतिः |
अनात्मनस्तु शत्रुत्वे वर्ते तात्मैव शत्रुवत् || 6||

bandhur ātmātmanas tasya yenātmaivātmanā jitaḥ
anātmanas tu śhatrutve vartetātmaiva śhatru-vat

'For those who have conquered the mind, it is their friend. For those who have failed to do so, the mind works like an enemy.'
– *Bhagavad Gita* (6:6) by Eknath Easwaran

This seventh limb, **dhyāna**, follows on closely from the sixth limb, **dhāraṇā** (concentration), in that we immerse ourselves in the object we have chosen to meditate on, transcending internal and external distractions. The only elements present in our awareness are ourselves and the object of meditation.

'tatra pratyaya-ikatanata dhyanam'

'An unbroken flow of knowledge to that object is Dhyana.'
– *The Yoga Sūtras of Patañjali* (3:2) by Swami Vivekananda

During this state of uninterrupted flow of thought, we become less aware of our surroundings and enter a calm, quiet and peaceful frame of mind. We become fully immersed in the present moment and can gain a greater sense of self-realisation and understanding for ourselves. There is no sense of judgement, no comparison and no analysis, just pure contentment. Connecting with ourselves at this level requires the practice of the previous limbs and a lot of patience.

14

Limb 8: Samādhi (pure awareness)

The final state of yoga is the eighth limb, known as **samādhi** (eternal bliss). This eighth limb of yoga helps us to explore the spiritual aspect of life.

As with Limb 7, this is not considered a 'practice' of yoga. Instead, it represents one of the highest states of meditation. At this stage, we no longer feel separate from the object of our meditation. It's like merging with it completely, where even the idea of 'meditating on something' starts to fade away. This is when we're fully absorbed in a deeper level of awareness.

During this state, we experience complete concentration and a deep sense of self-realisation. **Samādhi** can occur at certain moments or extend over longer periods. When we are in this state, we feel an intense connection to everything around us, and all worries and distractions simply fade away. Sounds blissful, right?

That's because it is! Imagine cultivating a state where you're fully present and unaffected by anything and everything. Your vision is clear, and you break free from the cycle of **saṃsāra** (as discussed on p. 79), liberating yourself from suffering and embracing deep and lasting joy and freedom. Ultimately, **samādhi** is believed to be the key to **mokṣa** (liberation) and inner peace.

Samādhi transcends ego, allowing us to connect with the highest levels of spiritual realisation. However, it is a deeply personal and subjective experience. Achieving **samādhi** requires dedicated and sincere meditation practice. Some individuals even devote their entire lives to working towards this state. It is not something that we can rush to and, as you've discovered, the previous limbs of yoga (and every aspect of this tradition) serve as stepping stones on this lifelong journey.

Saṃyama (the concept of combining Limbs 6–8)

The last three limbs of yoga – **dhāraṇā** (concentration), **dhyāna** (meditation) and **samādhi** (eternal bliss) can be merged for simplicity, and we call this concept **saṃyama**. The *Yoga Sūtras of Patañjali* (see p. 85) introduce us to the three final limbs in this combined way, and this approach can enrich our meditation experience and make it more accessible, too. For example, in this form, we can see the steps as follows:

- In the initial stage of **dhāraṇā**, we select an object, concept or idea to focus our attention on. Our goal is to concentrate on this point of focus as intensely as possible. While external distractions may occasionally take our focus away, we can train our minds to return to the object.
- As we progress into **dhyāna**, we find ourselves becoming absorbed in the chosen object. Distractions begin to fade, and the only elements present in our awareness are ourselves and the object of meditation.
- Lastly, we arrive at **samādhi**, which is the peak of meditative states. At this stage, the boundaries between ourselves and the object completely dissolve. It's a state where the distinction between the object and the act of meditation itself disappears. It's here that we are fully immersed in an elevated state of awareness.

Understanding this concept should hopefully provide you with a bit more clarity on your meditation journey. Remember, it's a gradual process where each step brings you closer to the higher states of consciousness that yoga offers.

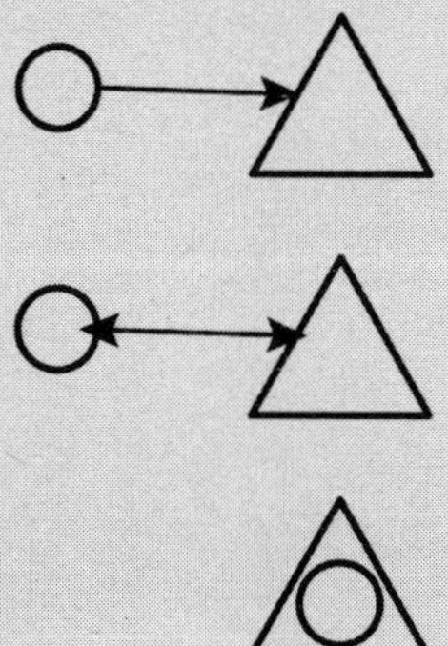

A moment of introspection

Now that we have come to the end of the eight limbs of yoga, take some time to sit with everything you have learned about **Aṣṭāṅga** yoga in its entirety.

We unpacked quite a lot! It might be worth thinking about what you might want to explore further or what you feel is most important for you to work on. Below are some questions to help you reflect:

- What aspects of the eight limbs of yoga were new and interesting for you?
- What's the most surprising thing you've discovered about the eight limbs of yoga?
- Do you believe that understanding the eight limbs of yoga will influence your current practice? If yes, how?
- Which of the eight limbs of yoga resonated with you the most? What's one simple step you could take from this limb to incorporate into your practice today?

15

Yoga Nidrā: a practice for deep relaxation

Yoga Nidrā is a practice of deep relaxation, which is often referred to as 'yogic sleep'. Its purpose is to promote deep rest and the release of physical, mental and emotional tension through inducing a state of relaxation. It is an accessible practice for people of all levels, particularly beginners.

Yoga Nidrā involves various practices aimed at deep relaxation and inner exploration. It includes visualisation, where you imagine images or scenarios; breath awareness, focusing on your breath pattern; awareness of sensations, noticing how your body feels; **sankalpas** (intentions), establishing positive affirmations or goals; and a conscious focus on thoughts or feelings. The technique of **Yoga Nidrā** is considered an evolution for the mind because it facilitates rapid learning and self-discovery. Our minds are very receptive, and we are therefore more inclined to absorb information while in a relaxed state, which is why **Yoga Nidrā** is so effective.

Typically, this practice is guided by an instructor, as verbal instructions are more effective during the experience. Unlike hypnosis, where direct commands are given, the instructions of **Yoga Nidrā** serve as gentle guidance, allowing you to explore your inner world freely. When practising **Yoga Nidrā**, you are advised to try to maintain awareness and not to fall asleep, but if you do that's also perfectly OK.

As per yogic traditions, the state we end up in during a **Yoga Nidrā** practice is where our true Self lies. If you haven't ever tried a **Yoga Nidrā** practice, I would highly recommend you do! Sometimes we can underestimate the importance of relaxation techniques, but this one in particular will give you great results when it comes to freeing the body of tension.

Benefits of Yoga Nidrā

- **Stress reduction** – **Yoga Nidrā** has been proven to be effective in regulating the nervous system and it is highly effective in managing stress and anxiety.
- **Improved sleep** – It can help with insomnia and sleep quality.
- **Focus** – The practice can help to bring you mental clarity and focus.
- **Creativity** – It can enhance your creativity.
- **Healing** – We can heal ourselves – physically, mentally and emotionally – through regular practice.

To practise

As I explained, this practice is typically guided by an instructor so to practise, simply scan the QR code provided in the Resources on p. 227. It will take you to a 10-minute **Yoga Nidrā** practice on my YouTube channel.

16

Studying yogic texts/ scriptures

Now that you're acquainted with yoga practices, let's explore another way to enrich your yoga journey. Often overlooked in modern yoga is the study of yogic texts (and this can lead to some of the issues with yoga today that we discussed in **Part 1**). However, if we connect our practice back to **svādhyāya** (self-study, see p. 161), it becomes very clear why delving into these texts is key for your path.

Svādhyāya encourages us to explore the classical texts, which hold such profound wisdom, and which we touched on in **Part 2** (see p. 82). By engaging in this study your understanding of spiritual practices will deepen and you'll help preserve yoga's traditions authentically, too. In this chapter, I'll be guiding you through how to approach these yoga texts and how they can help you cultivate a genuine yoga practice.

A **Yogaśāstra** is the name given to any yogic text or scripture that provides us with guidance on how to practise and study yoga. They include texts and scriptures that have been passed down through generations and that have influenced the development of yoga. In today's world, you'll often find translations of these texts from the Sanskrit language. Some of the most popular **Yogaśāstras** are the following (many of which we've touched on already, and which are listed in full on p. 228):

- *Bhagavad Gita*
- *Upanishads*
- *The Yoga Sūtras of Patañjali*
- *Haṭha Yoga Pradīpikā*
- *Gheranda Samhita*
- *Yoga Yājñavalkya*
- *Shiva Samhita*

Every **Yogaśāstra** is seen as a valuable resource for anyone who is pursuing the path of yoga as they detail the philosophy, principles and practices of yoga in its most traditional form. Each text has a different theme, but all of them have the purpose of helping us to gain yogic knowledge and wisdom to reach **mokṣa** (enlightenment).

For a beginner, exploring the **Yogaśāstras** may seem intimidating or confusing, especially without the guidance of a guru. So here are a few things to keep in mind when approaching your learning of the texts/scriptures.

1. **Understand your reasons for wanting to learn the text/scriptures** - Some people want to gain a deeper knowledge of the practice, some want to gain spiritual insights, and some want to learn more for personal growth. Whatever the purpose of your interest, being clear will help guide what you study and keep you motivated through the process.
2. **Seek guidance from a teacher or a mentor** - As a reminder, trying to decipher texts on your own can be difficult. Having someone who has studied the path of yoga and who has experience to help will enable you to learn things that you might not have discovered on your own. While it's best to learn from a teacher, translations can still be helpful if that's not possible.
3. **Study multiple translations or commentaries** - This will ensure that you have different perspectives, which can make learning easier. For example, I have read three different translations of the *Bhagavad Gita*, which helped me to write this book. I found the first translation too difficult to understand (even with the help of my teacher). It was only after reading a couple more translations that the first one made sense!
4. **Take notes** - As you may have been doing while reading this book, write down any reflections or key concepts that resonate with you as you go. This will help you to remember what you have learned so you can then integrate it into your life and practice.
5. **Establish a regular routine** - In yogic terms, we call this **sādhanā** or daily spiritual practice. Even dedicating just 10 minutes a day to this can make a big difference in the long run.
6. **Practise, practise, practise** - The only way to see or feel results is to stay consistent with your practice. Applying everything you have learned and observing how it has impacted your life is essential on the path of self-discovery.

The layout of scriptures – a case study

We won't have space to go through every **Yogaśāstra** here, but when it comes to studying the texts, you will notice that each one has its own unique layout. To give you a taster of what you can expect, and for the purpose of keeping it simple here, I'll describe the layout of one of the most common **Yogaśāstras**: *The Yoga Sūtras of Patañjali*. This text is among the most popular in modern yoga and is recommended on teacher training courses. It's considered the most accessible text (so it's one I suggest you start with), yet often practitioners struggle with how to use it effectively. We'll go through the structure together now so that if you'd like to explore *The Yoga Sūtras of Patañjali* further, you can use this as a guide.

The *Yoga Sūtras* are made up of four **pādas** (chapters or books).

Book 1: 'Samadhi Pāda' – the foundations of yoga

This foundational section of the text comprises of 51 **sūtras**, which are concise, memorable verses outlining key concepts of yoga. These include insights into the obstacles encountered in the practice, the goal of **Kriyā** yoga (see p. 116) and the importance of meditation. Every **sūtra** is concise and often easy to understand, making it simple to integrate into daily life. You can focus on one or two **sūtras** at a time, and there's no pressure to learn them all at once

One crucial **sūtra** - *'yogaś-citta-vrtti-nirodhah'* or 'Yoga is restraining the mind-stuff (Chitta) from taking various forms (Vrttis)' - emphasises restraining the fluctuations of the mind. By restraining these fluctuations, often referred to as **chitta vrittis**, we can attain a state of mental clarity and calmness, which allows us to focus more effectively during meditation and other aspects of yoga. Or, in Chapter 3, Verses 16 and 17, the concept of **saṃyama** (see p. 209), consisting of three stages, is outlined, providing further depth to the practice. This chapter also includes helpful lists to aid us in understanding the teachings, such as a list of the five **vrittis**, which represent different states of mental activity along with guidance on overcoming them. Beginners can access these teachings through books, online courses or by seeking guidance from experienced practitioners.

NOTES ON APPLYING THE TEACHINGS OF 'SAMADHI PĀDA'

- Begin a simple meditation routine.
- Practise mindfulness in your everyday activities, paying attention to your thoughts and emotions.
- Learn about how the mind works and how it changes.

Book 2: 'Sādhanā Pāda' – the eight limbs of yoga

The 55 **sūtras** included in this **pāda** focus on the practical aspects of yoga and this is where **Aṣṭāṅga** is described. Patañjali details the eight limbs and provides us with guidance on each one. He also shares the five **kleshas** (causes of suffering): **avidyā** (ignorance), **asmitā** (ego), **rāga** (attachment), **dveṣa** (aversion) and **abhiniveṣa** (fear of death). Following this, he provides us with a solution for each one.

NOTES ON APPLYING THE TEACHINGS OF 'SĀDHANĀ PĀDA'

- Embrace the teachings of **Aṣṭāṅga** yoga, which outlines the eight-limbed path (see p. 150).
- Develop a regular **āsana** (physical posture) and **prāṇāyāma** (breath control) practice.
- Study the ethical principles of **Aṣṭāṅga** (the **yamas** and **niyamas**, see p. 162).

Book 3: 'Vibhuti Pāda' – the supernatural powers of yoga

The third **pāda** includes 56 **sūtras** about **siddhis** (supernatural powers) that can be attained through yoga. These include powers such as telepathy and clairvoyance. Patañjali tells us that these powers come with the practise of advanced stages of yoga. He also emphasises the importance of not letting these powers distract us from our goal of self-realisation.

NOTES ON APPLYING THE TEACHINGS OF 'VIBHUTI PĀDA'

- Remember, the aim of yoga is to achieve **mokṣa**, not just to gain supernatural powers.
- Understand that while these **siddhis** can be fascinating, they're not the main focus of yoga. Instead, they naturally come as a bonus when you practise regularly and with dedication.

Book 4: 'Kaivalya Pāda' – liberation and self-realisation through yoga

The final **Pāda** teaches us the concept of the state of liberation and self-realisation through its 34 **sūtras**. Here, Patañjali discusses the nature of a liberated soul and how to achieve complete detachment from the material world, which he describes as **kaivalya**.

The concepts of **puruṣa** (true Self) and **prakṛti** (the material world) (see p. 112) are also introduced here. Patañjali helps us to explore our inner essence and understand our true nature. By understanding these ideas, we're guided towards uncovering a deep sense of peace within ourselves, ultimately leading to inner freedom.

NOTES ON APPLYING THE TEACHINGS OF 'KAIVALYA PĀDA'

- The aim is to achieve **kaivalya** or liberation and understand **saṃsāra** (the cycle of birth, death and rebirth). Find more on **saṃsāra** on p. 79.
- Consider how **puruṣa** is separate from **prakṛti**.
- Cultivate **bhakti** practice for liberation. Find more on **bhakti** on p. 123.

The purpose of this **Yogaśāstra** is to provide a guide to the philosophy of yoga that includes insights into the path of self-realisation, the eight limbs and the goal of **mokṣa**. This was just a brief introduction to *The Yoga Sūtras of Patañjali* but remember, every little step counts. So, take your time and enjoy exploring each part at your own pace.

Part Four

Continuing your journey

What now? Well, it's time to continue your practice in real time! It goes without saying that we've covered a great deal of information in this book, and for me to expect you to turn your practice around or implement everything that we have spoken about instantly would be unrealistic. As I mentioned throughout, my intention when I began this book was to give you information to guide you towards a well-rounded and authentic practice that feels right for you. I hope this has remained clear for you while reading this, and that you've enjoyed your learning so far. In this section I offer some advice on where to go next as well as my hope for the future of the modern yoga practice.

Ten next steps

If you need a little inspiration on where to go next, here are some steps that will help you to continue in a respectful way. Remember, even taking just one of these steps is better than doing nothing. Focus on one step at a time...

1. **Continue learning and educating yourself** – Investing time to learning the background, roots and history of the ancient practice of yoga will ensure you benefit from it in the best way possible.

   This might look like looking back through **Part 2** and choosing a part of yoga's history to look further into or picking a yoga text to read.

2. **Seek out authentic sources** – This includes books, teachers and online sources. Always look for teachings or practices that have cultural significance.

   This might look like following authentic teachers on social media (you can find some on p. 226) who have a deep understanding of yoga and its cultural roots. When seeking information, opt for sources that draw from traditional yoga texts (similar to the ones we discussed in **Part 2**) or are recommended by trusted experts. Or it could be selecting a space for your yoga practice that truly captures the essence of (authentic) yoga (see guidance for this on p. 137).

3. **Find your community** – Connect with people and spaces that highlight the cultural, spiritual and philosophical elements of yoga, and who teach yoga from an informed perspective.

   This might look like having conversations with other teachers and practitioners. Browse the resources section of this book or look up yoga teachers in your area and choose ones that align with you, and practise with them.

4. **Support inclusivity and accessibility** – Uplift voices and spaces that advocate for inclusivity and choose environments where yoga is accessible for everybody regardless of race, body type or abilities.

   This might look like engaging with yoga teachers and environments that make everyone feel included and seeking out spaces where yoga is accessible to everyone, as we discussed in **Part 1.**

5. **Encourage others to explore authentic yoga** – Share your journey and insights of yoga and let others know that yoga has many more aspects to it beyond the physical. Advocate for authenticity and inspire others to do the same.

   This might look like speaking about your journey within your community. Or buying a book like this one for a friend or for anyone who is interested in beginning yoga but doesn't know where to start. Another idea is to lend your copy of this book to a friend and then have a chat about it afterwards.

6. **Be mindful of trends and commercialisation** – Avoid trends and brands that encourage gimmicky types of yoga.

   This might look like sidestepping brands that appropriate or disrespect the practice of yoga. Be mindful of not practising with puppies, wine or goats, or taking part in any other novelty types of yoga. Using the reflective questions in **Parts 1** and **2** may also help you to be mindful of practising yoga respectfully.

7. **Implement the teachings of yoga in everyday life** – As you now know, yoga can be applied in various aspects of life. Stay committed to yoga as a path of self-realisation.

   This might look like picking a practice from this book to apply to your daily life. Use the practices in **Part 3** to help you stay committed to using yoga as a tool for self-growth and self-development.

8. **Become comfortable with being uncomfortable** – Yoga isn't always about feeling good; it involves ups and downs, highs and lows. Embrace and accept that there will be discomfort.

   This might look like sticking to a routine for your practice even when your life gets busy. Remember **tapas** (the willingness to endure discomfort for a higher purpose, see p. 160)! You may also find reminding yourself of the nine obstacles in yoga (see p. 110) helpful. Understanding these can help you accept that your practice won't always look perfect and that's absolutely fine.

9. **Create room for reflection** – As you've practised yoga through reading and engaging with this book, ensure you consistently reflect on and are introspective about new insights. This ongoing self-awareness aligns with the essence of yoga.

   This might look like regularly journalling or opening up to a friend or family member who you feel safe around. Continuing to ask yourself questions similar to our 'Moments of introspection' that you've already been practising may also be beneficial in understanding yourself and your practice.

10. **Question and be mindful** – Become inquisitive when it comes to practices that don't look like they align with the traditional teachings of yoga. If you see spaces where the roots are disregarded or disrespected, question their authenticity. Refer to **Part 1** to help you.

    This might look like reaching out to teachers or studios if you notice their practices aren't aligned with authentic yoga teachings. While it may feel daunting and might not always be well-received, expressing your concerns respectfully can have a significant impact. I've personally experienced instances where people were open to receiving feedback about practising yoga authentically.

2

My hope for the future

When I began raising awareness around the lack of authenticity in yoga in the Western world, I never imagined that it would be possible to make a change. However, as time went on and people like yourself began to support the work that I and other native teachers do, I realised it *was* actually possible. Five years down the line of doing this work, I have seen significant changes, even if we do still have a long way to go! But here is a hopeful timeline of the changes that I wish to see in the yoga industry in the years to come. I'd love for us to work on this dream together.

Next few years - Get ready for more diversity, inclusivity and awareness in yoga. We'll see culturally significant classes and spaces where yoga is taught in its most authentic form with the teachings including more than physical poses. People will feel comfortable discussing the issues of Western yoga and will dig into the roots and history of yoga, embracing the often-overlooked elements.

Next 5 to 10 years - Brace yourself for widely recognised education standards in yoga and the establishment of an *official* governing board. Access to authentic yoga teacher trainings will expand globally. Yoga will gain recognition for its spiritual, mental and emotional benefits, outdoing its physical aspects. Expect to see the representation of BIPOC amplified in brands and spaces.

Beyond 10 years - The push to preserve the roots of yoga will increase. Social and economic barriers will dissolve, making yoga accessible to everyone. As yoga adapts to modern societal needs, these modifications will be made with the highest respect. Get ready for a world of yoga that truly serves and benefits everyone!

Final thoughts

> 'The Self cannot be found in books.
> You have to find it for yourself in yourself.'
>
> Ramana Maharshi

These words beautifully encapsulate the essence of my intentions in writing this book. I hope this book has served as a guide, helping you to explore yourself through the less commonly studied practices of yoga in the modern day.

Although there is *so* much more that can be said on every topic in this book, it is intended for any seeker on the yogic path. Whether your goal is healing through yoga, teaching it or simply gaining more knowledge on the topic, I hope that it has planted seeds for the many ways yoga can benefit you.

Writing this book has been an incredibly challenging journey for me. It required deep thought for every sentence. (And considering that I don't come from a writing background and left university after the first year – for fear of writing essays! – it was no easy task.) I hope you can recognise the effort it took to articulate and put my thoughts on to paper, as it demanded everything from me to reach this point. Throughout the process, I faced three major episodes of depression, several occurrences of burnout, left my full-time job and grappled daily with my mental health at the same time as trying to work on my business. Yoga got me through a lot of these difficult periods, and I hope it does the same for you, too.

Despite the challenges, 2023 and 2024 were years of reflection and introspection. Although I struggled, I managed to pick myself up enough to complete the task of writing this book. My greatest hope is that it positively impacts your practice and the world of yoga for years to come. Thank you for reaching this point and for your efforts in reclaiming the authenticity of yoga. Your journey is truly valued.

Resources

Yoga teacher trainings, workshops, retreats and courses

Arya Yoga Studio (www.aryayogastudio.com): Online membership, classes and workshops by Nikita Desai.

Arhanta Yoga (www.arhantayoga.org): A yoga training institute established by Ram Jain.

Kaivalyadhama (www.kdham.com): Yoga education, online courses, workshops and research.

Yoga Prasad Institute (www.yogaprasad.in): Online yoga courses, teacher training and workshops by yoga educator Prasad Rangnekar.

Svastha (www.svastha.net): Yoga education and online learning founded by A. G. Mohan and Indra Mohan.

Act Yoga (www.actyoga.in): Teacher training retreats and videos by yoga instructor Dr Ganesh Rao.

Find Your Breath (www.findyourbreath.net): Yoga retreats, courses and online membership by Melissa Shah.

Yog Sadhna (www.yogsadhna.com): Mentoring, training and retreats by Indu Arora.

Wandering Mat (www.wanderingmat.com): Retreats and courses by Vikramjeet Singh.

ABCD Yogi (www.abcdyogi.com): Online yoga community, courses and classes centred around uplifting South Asian teachers and marginalised groups by Tejal Patel.

The Yoga Institute (www.theyogainstitute.org): Teacher training, classes, courses and workshops by Dr Hansaji.

Useful yoga websites

Yoga Sequence Builder (www.tummee.com): A yoga sequencing builder app/ site that has an endless amount of information on yogic practices including **āsana** and **prāṇāyāma**. This site also has voice notes for the pronunciation of Sanskrit terms.

Vivekavani (www.vivekavani.com): A collection of yoga quotes, topics and texts that includes commentary on core yogic texts such as the *Bhagavad Gita*.

The following QR codes will take you to a **7 Days of Yoga for Beginners** programme and a **Yoga Nidrā** practice on my YouTube channel (@Nikyyoga):

7 Days of Yoga for Beginners

Yoga Nidrā

YouTube

- Nikyyoga (@Nikyyoga)
- Ventuno Yoga (@VentunoYoga)
- The Sanskrit Channel (@TheSanskritChannel)
- Satvic Movement (@SatvicMovement)
- Arhanta Yoga (@Arhanta_Yoga)
- Tejal Yoga (@TejalYoga)
- Sanskriti Yoga (@mahavenk)
- Yogaprasad Institute (@Yogaprasad)
- The Yoga Institute (@theyogainstituteofficial)
- Prashantj Yoga (@Prashantj Yoga)

Podcasts

'Let's Talk Yoga' by Arundhati Baitmangalkar (https://letstalk.yoga)

'Yoga is Dead' by Tejal Patel and Jesal Parikh (www.yogaisdeadpodcast.com/about-us)

Bibliography

Bhattacharya, Dr Bhaswati, *Everyday Ayurveda: Daily Habits That Can Change Your Life in a Day* (Random House India, 2019)

Chandra Vasu, Srisa, *The Shiva Samhita* (Apurva Krishna Bose, Indian Press, 1914)

Charaka, Acharya, *Charaka Samhita: handbook on ayurveda* (independently published, 2016)

Desikachar, T. K. V., *The Heart of Yoga* (Inner Traditions, 1995)

Easwaran, Eknath, *The Bhagavad Gita* (Nilgiri Press, 2007)

Easwaran, Eknath, *The Upanishads* (Nilgiri Press, 2007)

Lad, Vasant, *The Complete Book of Ayurvedic Home Remedies* (Platkus, 2006)

Mohan, A. G., *Yoga for the Body, Breath, and Mind* (Shambhala Publications Inc, 1993)

Mohan, A. G, Mohan, Ganesh, *Yoga Yājñavalkya,* (Svastha Yoga Pte, 2013)

Muktibodhananda, Swami, *Haṭha Yoga Pradīpikā* (Bihar School of Yoga, India, 1998)

Saraswati, Swami Niranjananda, *Gheranda Samhita* (Bihar School of Yoga, 2012)

Saraswati, Swami Satyananada, *Asana Pranayama Mudra Bandha* (Bihar School of Yoga, 2013)

Sastry, Trilochan, *The Essentials of Hinduism* (Penguin Random House India, 2022)

Singleton, M., *Roots of Yoga* (Penguin Random House UK, 2017)

Singleton, M., *Yoga Body: The Origins of Modern Posture Practice* (Oxford University Press, USA, 2010).

Sivananda, Swami, *Bhagavad Gita* (The Divine Life Trust Society, World Wide Web Edition, 2000)

Sivananda, Swami, *The Science of Pranayama* (Divine Life Society, 2009)

Swami, Om, *Kuṇḍalinī, An Untold Story* (Jaico Publishing House 2016)

Swatmarama, Swami (translated by Pancham Sinh), *Haṭha Yoga Pradīpikā* (CreateSpace Independent Publishing Platform, 2011)

Vaughn, Amy, *From the Vedas to Vinyasa* (Opening Lotus Publications, 2016)

Vivekananda, Swami, *Bhakti Yoga: The Yoga of Love and Devotion* (Advaita Ashrama, 2010)

Vivekananda, Swami, *Jnana Yoga: The Yoga of Knowledge* (Vedānta Press, 1998)

Vivekananda, Swami, *Karma Yoga: The Yoga of Action* (independently published, 2020)

Vivekananda, Swami, *Raja Yoga* (Advaita Ashrama, 2017)

Vivekananda, Swami, *The Yoga Sūtras of Patañjali* (Fingerprint! Classics, 2023)

Yogananda, Paramahansa, *Autobiography of a Yogi* (Self Realization Fellowship, 2019)

References

How to use this book

'Books are infinite in number, and time is short; therefore, this is the secret of knowledge, to take that which is essential': Vivekananda, Swami, *The Yoga Sūtras of Patañjali* (Fingerprint! Classics, 2023).

A note on sanskrit

'Sanskrit is a phonetic language and gives much importance to accents, pitch and pronunciation': S Satchidananda, Swami, *The Yoga Sūtras of Patanjali* (Integral Yoga Publications, 2015)

Part 1

1. Problem 1: The emphasis on physicality in modern yoga

'Swami Jnaneshvara Bharati, who said that it's false to think "yoga is a physical system with a spiritual component"': www.swamij.com/traditional-yoga.htm

'In 2019, the *Daily Telegraph* shed light on this concerning trend': 'Instagram is fuelling [a] rise in injuries among yoga teachers who want [the]

perfect social media post"': Lyons, I. *The Daily Telegraph*, 3 November 2019 [Online].

2. Problem 2: Cultural appropriation in modern yoga

'Cultural appropriation': Britannica. Available at: www.britannica.com/story/what-is-cultural-appropriation

'A recent article in the *Guardian* raised concerns on young puppies being unfairly treated as working animals': '"Puppy yoga" is on the rise – and as a dog welfare specialist, I'm horrified', Wheeler, Esme, the *Guardian*, 13 July 2023 [Online].

4. Problem 4: The lack of diversity in modern yoga

'a 2019 study, which analysed the coverage of yoga and accessibility within mainstream yoga': 'Yoga is for Every (Able) Body: A Content Analysis of Disability Themes within Mainstream Yoga Media', Thomas, V., Warren-Findlow, J. and Webb, J., *International Journal of Yoga,* January-April 2019. Available at: www.ncbi.nlm.nih.gov/pmc/articles/PMC6329228/

'Rebekah Boatrite said: "Our communities are the reflection..."': 'Anti-Racism and Representation in Yoga and Wellness Spaces', Boatrite, R., *Vesselify*. Available at: https://vesselify.com/2020/06/anti-racism-and-representation-in-yoga-and-wellness-spaces/

Part 2

1. A brief timeline of the history of yoga

'Disclaimer: Pinpointing exact dates is challenging': Sastry, Trilochan, *The Essentials of Hinduism* (Penguin Random House India, 2022)

4. Significant gurus of yoga

'He describes Kriya yoga as "an instrument through which human evolution can be quickened"': Yogananda, Paramahansa, *Autobiography of a Yogi*, (Self-Realization Fellowship, 1998)

'his guru told him: "I want you to enter college in Calcutta ... Hindu teacher has a university degree."': Yogananda, Paramahansa, *Autobiography of a Yogi*, (Self-Realization Fellowship, 1998)

'His teachings were mostly based on *The Yoga Sūtras of Patañjali* (p. 85) and the *Yoga Yājñavalkya*': Mohan, A. G, Mohan, Ganesh, *Yoga Yājñavalkya,* (Svastha Yoga Pte, 2013)

Part 3

1. Three key yogic teachings

'Lord Krishna reassures Arjuna that the restless mind can be controlled by a dedicated practice': https://vivekavani.com/b6v35/

'It is true that the mind is restless and difficult to control. But it can be conquered, Arjuna through regular practice and detachment.': Easwaran, Eknath, *Bhagavad Gita* (6:35) (Nilgiri Press, 2007).

'Persevere. All progress proceeds by rise and fall': Vivekananda, Swami, *The Yoga Sūtras of Patañjali* (1:30) (Fingerprint! Classics, 2023)

'Purusa is that part of us capable of real seeing and perception. It is not subject to change. Conversely, Prakrti is subject to constant change and embraces all matter, even our mind, thoughts, feelings, and memories.': Desikachar, T. K. V., *The Heart of Yoga* (Inner Traditions, 1999), p. 94.

3. Traditional yoga: the four key mārgas

'a study carried out in 2013 on the effects of Karma yoga ... a therapeutic method for reducing anxiety and stress': Kumar, Arun and Kumar, Sanjay, 'Karma yoga: A path towards work in positive psychology', *Indian Journal of Psychiatry*, 55(2), January 2013. Available at: www.ncbi.nlm.nih.gov/pmc/articles/PMC3705674/

'This short quote from the *Gita* sums up Karma yoga': https://vivekavani.com/b3v19/

'Therefore, without attachment, do thou always perform action which should be done; for, by performing action without attachment man reaches the Supreme.': Sivananda, Swami, *Bhagavad Gita* (3:19) (The Divine Life Trust Society, World Wide Web Edition, 2000)

'This is reflected in the *Bhagavad Gita* as Lord Krishna says the following': https://vivekavani.com/b12v2/

'Those who set their hearts on me and worship me with unfailing devotion and faith are more established in yoga': Easwaran, Eknath, *Bhagavad Gita* (12:2) (Nilgiri Press, 2007).

'With senses and mind constantly controlled through meditation, united with the Self within, an aspirant attains nirvana, the state of abiding joy and peace in me.': Easwaran, Eknath, *Bhagavad Gita* (6:15) (Nilgiri Press, 2007).

'Take time to discover your guru or teacher': https://vivekavani.com/b4v34/

'Approach those who have realized the purpose of life and question them with reverence and devotion; they will instruct you in this wisdom.' – *Bhagavad Gita* (4:34) by Eknath Easwaran

4. Traditional yoga: Haṭha yoga

'A yogi should have a free and open mind': Muktibodhananda, Swami, *Haṭha Yoga Pradīpikā* (Bihar School of Yoga, India, 1998).

'Even the daily act of cleaning purifies the mind': Muktibodhananda, Swami, *Haṭha Yoga Pradīpikā* (Bihar School of Yoga, India, 1998), p. 44.

'There are other benefits, too, as it can balance the hormones, purify the nervous system and reduce symptoms of depression.': 'Nauli Kriya: Detoxifying Inner Anatomy and Physiology,' Rathod, Kushal Hon., *International Journal of Science and Research*, 5 May 2023. Available at: https://www.ijsr.net/archive/v12i5/SR23523092542.pdf

'Being the first accessory of Haṭha yoga, āsana is described first. It should be practised for gaining steady posture, health, and lightness of the body.': Swatmarama, Swami (translated by Pancham Sinh), *Haṭha Yoga Pradīpikā* (Pacific Publishing Studio, 2011), p. 6.

'When the body is overloaded with food, it becomes sluggish, and the mind becomes dull': Muktibodhananda, Swami, *Haṭha Yoga Pradīpikā* (Bihar School of Yoga, India, 1998), p. 44.

'Although many Āyurvedic rituals can take weeks, months or sometimes even years to work, many studies show that the benefits and effects are profound.' 'Are ayurveda treatments and ayurvedic medicine effective? Ask the Professor, with SCU's Dr. Anu', Kizhakkeveettil, Anupama, Southern California University of Health Studies. Available at: https://www.scuhs.edu/front-page-news/atp-efficacy-of-ayurveda/

'Gandusha – Oil pulling involves holding oil in the mouth for a period of time to promote gut health and prevent diseases of the mouth.' 'Kavala and Gandusha – Need for Oral Health', Najma Sultana, K.J and Katti, Anand, *International Journal of Ayurveda and Pharmaceutical Chemistry,* 10 March 2022. Available at: http://ijapc.com/upload/MNAPC-16-I2-(v16-i1-16)-P-173-182.pdf

'Jihwa prakṣālana – Removing toxins from the body by gently scraping the tongue. This also helps improve the digestive system.': 'Tongue Scraping – Jihwa Prakshalana', Buddhist Studies Institute. Available at: https://buddhistudiesinstitute.org/courses/simple-dinacharya/lessons/tongue-scraping-jihwa-prakshalana/

9. Limb 3: Āsana (physical postures)

'it's advised to practise Vajrāsana after meals as it is believed to improve digestion,': 'The influence of Vajrasana (thunderbolt pose) on an individual', Naragatti, Siddappa and Hosakote, Vadiraja S, *Global Journal for Research Analysis* 12(9):1-6, September 2023.

'The distance between the feet … allowing the fingers to curl slightly.': Saraswati, Swami Niranjananda, *Gheranda Samhita* (Bihar School of Yoga, 2012), p. 204.

10. Limb 4: Prāṇāyāma (regulation of breath)

'Swami Sivananda articulates this in his book *The Science of Pranayama* where he writes: "Prana becomes visible on the physical plane as motion and action, and on the mental plane as thought."': Sivananda, Swami, *The Science of Pranayama* (Divine Life Society, 2009)

'Physically, the practice of kumbhaka increases carbon dioxide in the body, which helps us to utilise the oxygen in our bodies over time.': 'The Immediate Effect of Yogasana On Oxygen Saturation Levels in Young Adults', Taru, Rutuja and Kaluskar, Rasika. Available at: http://210.212.169.38/xmlui/handle/123456789/10095

11. Limb 5: Pratyāhāra (the influence of our senses)

'As T. K. V. Desikachar says, "Precisely because the mind is so focused, the senses follow it; it is not happening the other way around."': Desikachar, T. K. V., *The Heart of Yoga* (Inner Traditions, 1995)

'The drawing in of the organs is by their giving up their own objects and taking the form of the mind-stuff': Vivekananda, Swami, *The Yoga Sūtras of Patañjali* (2:54) (Fingerprint! Classics, 2023)

12. Limb 6: Dhāraṇā (concentration)

'Dhāraṇā (concentration) is when the mind holds on to some object, either in the body, or outside the body, and keeps itself in that state': Vivekananda, Swami, *The Yoga Sūtras of Patañjali* (3:1) (Fingerprint! Classics, 2023)

'Swami Swatmarama shares this practice with us and says: "the impression of the flame remains for some time"': Muktibodhananda, Swami, *Haṭha Yoga Pradīpikā* (Bihar School of Yoga, India, 1998).

13. Limb 7: Dhyāna (meditation)

'For those who have conquered the mind, it is their friend. For those who have failed to do so, the mind works like an enemy.': https://vivekavani.com/b6v6/

'An unbroken flow of knowledge to that object is Dhyana': Vivekananda, Swami, *The Yoga Sūtras of Patañjali* (3:2) (Fingerprint! Classics, 2023)

16. Studying yogic texts/scriptures

'Yoga is restraining the mind-stuff (Chitta) from taking various forms (Vrttis)': Vivekananda, Swami, *The Yoga Sūtras of Patañjali* (x:xx) (Fingerprint! Classics, 2023)

Acknowledgements

First and foremost, I express my deepest gratitude to God for blessing me with everything that I have and for shaping me into who I am. Embracing and appreciating myself has been a journey, and my faith has been a guiding light through life's challenges. I extend heartfelt thanks to my ancestors and every guru and teacher who contributed to shaping my practice, preserving our traditions and fighting the good fight.

I'd like to thank Bloomsbury for providing me with this opportunity to write my first book! A very special thank you to Holly Jarrald for finding my work through social media and seeing the potential in my work for this book to be shaped into what it is now. You have been so patient, understanding, helpful and supportive throughout this entire process. Thank you for understanding my ideas, for asking all the right questions and helping me to refine it over and over until it looked like this. Your feedback has taught me more than you know, and your guidance has been invaluable. I'd also like to thank Meg and Lucy for their invaluable contributions in bringing this book to its current standard. Meg, your assistance in answering my countless questions and helping with the intricate details has been incredibly helpful. Lucy, your thoroughness and attention to the smallest details ensured nothing was overlooked. Thank you to all the other teams at Bloomsbury for making this book everything I dreamed of.

Thank you to my family for your unwavering support. Without you, I wouldn't have been able to pursue the many dreams that I have, but especially not this one. Mama, you have always been there no matter what and your ability to love unconditionally has inspired me daily. Thank you for always being there at whatever time I need you and for keeping me well-fuelled with your delicious food every day! Thank you for the shoulder and neck massages after long days of writing! Papa, your love never fails to amaze me! Thank you for always showing up, and for helping me in every way you can to support my health, my career and every aspect of life. Your hard work and dedication are thought of every time things get tough for me. My sister, Bhav, thank you for being my pillar of strength and for lifting me out of every episode of depression. I couldn't ever thank you enough for everything you have done and continue to do for me. Thank you for teaching me some of my greatest lessons, for teaching me how to be graceful and kind and for being a source of inspiration every day of my life. Thank you for believing in me when I didn't believe in myself during the challenging moments of writing this book. Thank you to my brothers. Vish, thank you for being the best big brother, for always looking out for me and for supporting me in every way that you can. Sham, thank you for listening to me and hearing me. Your understanding has helped me through my best and worst times, thank you bestie! Thank you to my brother-in-law Tushar, and both my sister-in-laws Viral and Fefe for your many caring ways, for your love and thoughtfulness, I'm so lucky to have you. Thank you to my nieces (girlies) and nephew (my little man), your smiles brought joy to my long writing days. Kali and Rafiki, my fur babies, thank you for being my emotional support.

To my friends, there are so many of you who deserve a space here, but to keep it short I will specifically name a few who have played a pivotal role in my yoga journey. Derya, thank you for always being present from the beginning. Even though you live far away, I still feel your love and care through every interaction we have. Thank you for encouraging me to keep going even when I didn't want to. Nikita, thank you for being the most supportive, caring and understanding friend. You've been there for me during the many times when I've broken down while writing this book. Thank you for your genuine care and compassion and for helping me with certain elements of this book. Matt, if it wasn't for you, I am sure I wouldn't be writing this! Thank you for constantly nagging me to be consistent with TikTok! Thank you for always hearing me out, being there and giving me some of the most important advice that I will always cherish.

To all my friends who lift me up and encourage me to keep going, who celebrate me and who are consistently by my side, you know who you are. Thank you!

My heartfelt thanks to Vex and Kaushal. Thank you for being a big support throughout some of the most important parts of my career. Thank you Vex for taking the time to talk to me when I first received the offer for this book. I didn't know how to navigate the next steps and you helped me when I didn't know any other person in the industry to turn to. A huge thank you for writing the foreword for my first book! I don't think I would have had it any other way! Your writing has inspired me for years and years and your words have helped me to heal and have shaped me into the person I am today. Kaush, you're the sweetest soul I know, thank you for always encouraging me to teach and for uplifting my work in the many ways you have. I really value you and our friendship.

Thank you to my therapist, you have been a huge part of my life journey for 12 years! I have needed you the most throughout the years of writing this book and you've helped me to navigate some of my most turbulent times. Thank you for understanding me in ways I never thought anyone could and thank you for always being honest, kind and considerate.

Thank you to my teacher, Prasad Rangnekar, for being a great source of knowledge and for always advocating for authenticity in yoga. You have taught me so much and I am forever grateful for your wisdom and input throughout my journey.

For every single person who has uplifted my voice, bought this book, supported me on social media, followed my journey and allowed me to guide them through a class, to everyone who I have mentored, motivated or inspired, thank you from the bottom of my heart. Thank you to the incredibly strong people whose voices I have featured throughout this book, I appreciate your strength and time in sharing your stories. Thank you for my social media platforms, especially TikTok for making this journey possible. Without each and every one of you to support my work, spread the word and share my teachings this wouldn't be possible. Immense gratitude goes out to all of you. Thank you!

ॐ शान्तिः
Om śāntih

Index